Eczema Diet Cookbook

Charles Thompson

Copyright© 2020by Charles Thompson

Contents

Eczema Diet Cookbook

Introduction

Also classified, according to some taxonomies, like dermatitis, eczema is the most frequent non-contagious skin disease. Currently, the causes of eczema are still unclear. In this regard, the researchers hypothesized that both environmental and genetic factors play a determining role. It represents a particular way of the skin's reaction to various internal and external factors and is characterized by the presence of reliefs or vesicles, desquamation, itching, and redness. The size and the area in which the lesions appear on the skin are too varied, and the causes can determine them. There are many types of eczema, but, two main types can be distinguished:

- eczema caused by aggressive external (exogenous) factors
- eczema directly dependent on the body itself (endogenous)

In some cases, the two factors may be present simultaneously: for example, endogenous eczema can be aggravated by external factors such as direct skin contact with irritants (solvents, detergents). Sometimes two or more forms of eczema can appear simultaneously, complicating disease detection and treatment. The ailments' intensity and duration can also vary: from light and transient state to acute and/or chronic conditions with a period ranging from a few weeks to a few months or even years. Clearly, in the latter case, the manifestation of eczema does not have a continuous trend. Still, it alternates periods in which it is not present with others in which it appears again, often also based on the seasons. This is because changes in temperature and exposure to sunlight can act as flare-ups

Chapter 1: What is Eczema?

Eczema is the term by which doctors refer to inflammation of the skin (or skin), generally characterized by itching, erythema (i.e., redness), blistering, and/or crusting. There are several types of eczema; each has some particularities, which an expert eye can recognize.

ARE ECZEMA AND DERMATITIS SYNONYMOUS?

In medicine, the terms eczema and dermatitis are synonymous, so they refer to the skin's same inflammatory condition.

EPIDEMIOLOGY

According to some statistical surveys, the people worldwide who suffered from eczema in 2010 were about 230 million, or about 3.5% of the world population. Eczema mainly affects young people: for example, in the United Kingdom, about 20% of children suffer from dermatitis; in the United States, about 10%. The sex most affected is the female one. Curiously and for reasons still unclear, from 1940 to 2000, eczema's incidence rate has been increasing. In other words, over the years, eczema has become an increasingly common problem. An interesting US study from 2010 investigated how prevalent eczema was among individuals with a job in the United States that year. It found that dermatitis affected about 10% of workers (i.e., more than 15 million individuals) and was particularly prevalent among health and social workers.

Forms of eczema

Depending on the prevalence of one disorder (symptom) over the other, the causes and the affected area are different distinguished forms of eczema; the main ones are:

Atopic eczema: also known as atopic dermatitis, it is the most common form of eczema. It mainly affects children but can also appear in adolescents and adults with different characteristics depending on age.

It is often accompanied by allergic manifestations such as bronchial asthma and allergic rhinitis. Those affected are often sensitive to allergens (substances capable of triggering an allergy) of food origin (milk, egg, etc.) or present in the air (pollen, dust, feathers, etc.). Genetic or hereditary factors are also involved. Generally, the body's most affected parts are the knees, elbows, neck, hands, face, and scalp.

Contact eczema (or contact dermatitis): is a type of eczema that occurs when the body comes into contact with an irritant, usually of chemical origin. The most important sensitizing substances are made up of chromates, cobalt salts, formaldehyde, nickel, and manganese, often present in detergents and solvents also in everyday use. It can be of allergic or irritative origin. It occurs in the skin area that comes into contact with the triggering substance and, initially, remains confined to that area. Later, however, it can spread to other parts of the body.

Discoid eczema (or discoid dermatitis or nummular eczema): owes its name to the characteristic circular or oval shape of the patches that occur on the skin. The cause is unknown, although it is often associated with dry skin. It mainly affects adults between the ages of 50 and 70. The patches can appear anywhere on the body but, in particular, occur on the forearms, back, hands, or feet. The face and scalp are generally excluded.

Seborrheic eczema (or seborrheic dermatitis): it is manifested by red and scaly patches, combined with itching, well defined, and localized on the sides of the nose, eyebrows, ears, scalp, and back.

Dyshidrotic eczema (or Dyshidrotic dermatitis or pompholix): It is characterized by small itchy blisters located mainly on the palms of the hands or soles of the feet, often between the fingers. The causes are not sure but are associated with excessive sweating and metal allergy.

Varicose eczema: generally affecting the itchy legs and inflamed, scaly skin around areas with varicose veins. The main cause is the presence of varicose veins and poor blood circulation in the affected area.

Causes

The causes of eczema are often unknown; a wide variety of external and internal factors, acting individually or in combination, can cause it. In general, however, at birth, there is already a skin sensitivity that predisposes it to the onset of the disease. In cases of irritative and allergic contact eczema, the causes are found in the substances the body has come into contact with. Very often, this type of eczema depends on substances handled in the context of one's work (people involved in construction, in the chemical and textile industry, painters, hairdressers, bakers, and confectioners, etc.), so much so that it is often called "professional dermatitis. " It can also happen that the triggering cause is associated, over time, with sensitization of the skin, making the disease chronic.

Bacterial infections, mainly staphylococcal or streptococcal, or those caused by fungi, are very persistent in excoriated skin areas and cause secretions on the eczematous lesions. The causes are attributable to the germs present. Infectious eczema is often a complication of other types of eczema. About eczema that develops from internal causes, it is more difficult to analyze its origin. Various genetic, immunological, and environmental factors are involved; even stress seems to be a trigger.

In summary, the causes can be of type:

- allergic
- irritative
- infectious
- genetic
- from stress

The condition tends to worsen with exposure to certain risk factors:

- pollen
- molds
- dust mites
- animals
- certain foods (for allergic individuals)
- some medications
- cold and dry air
- contact with irritating chemicals
- direct skin contact with natural (wool) or synthetic raw fabrics
- additives found in soaps and skin lotions

Chapter 2: Symptoms and Complications

Symptoms

Given the great variety of eczema, the disorders (symptoms) they cause can also be very different. However, some disorders are always present that can combine by varying in intensity and rapidity of onset. The predominant condition in all forms of eczema is itching combined with blisters (small pads of the skin containing serous fluid) which, over time, due to their rubbing, tend to break. The vesicles' rupture causes the outflow of the liquid contained in them and the formation of small crusts of a generally round shape. In eczema forms that appear suddenly and rapidly (acute), the scabs are usually more extensive.

In the phase preceding the healing, small scales gradually diminish until they disappear (total recovery). In some cases, the healing process can be interrupted by a relapse (flare-up).

The different phases of eczema can alternate with each other and be present simultaneously in different areas of the body.

Another often characteristic element of eczema is dry and red skin.

In summary, the major disorders (symptoms) caused by eczema are:

- itch
- redness
- appearance of blisters
- appearance of crusts
- desquamation

The itching can be of varying intensity; in some cases, it can even be so intense and long-lasting that it interferes with the quality of life by causing insomnia, lack of appetite, and nervousness.

Duration of symptoms

Eczema can occur in a mild and transient form or an acute and transient form, or even in a chronic form. In the latter case, the duration of the symptoms fluctuates between a few weeks and a few months; it can last for years in some patients. The chronic forms do not have a continuous course but alternate periods of symptom remission with periods in which these, due to seasonal changes or sudden temperature changes, reappear.

Complications

Scratching and rubbing induced by itching and discomfort caused by skin lesions may themselves be at the root of bruises and scratches. These represent breaches in the skin through which germs of various types can enter, responsible for skin infections that can spread to the underlying tissue and adjacent lymph nodes. The so-called infectious eczema is often a complication of other types of eczema. Staphylococci or streptococci mainly cause bacterial infections. Viral infections can lead to the formation of warts or the appearance of the so-called molluscum contagiosum, transmissible skin infection due to a Poxvirus that causes pink or white formation dome-shaped growths. When a fungus is responsible for the infection, the skin is easily bruised.

Psychological factor

The intense itching caused by eczema can limit patients' quality of life by reducing the quality of sleep (penalized by frequent awakenings and restlessness), a continuous feeling of nervousness and irritability, and a sense of social inadequacy. Like all dermatological pathologies, it affects an organ, the skin, which represents the barrier that separates us from the outside world. Especially when the symptoms appear on the face, the disease has a decisive impact on interpersonal relationships. The situation can be particularly problematic when the patient is pediatric. Skin manifestations and itching make eczema potentially disabling in school placement and relationships with peers. The problem is all the more complicated, the more the vicious circle is established in which the disease produces psychological malaise, which triggers or worsens states of psychophysical and emotional tension, exacerbating the symptoms and, in fact, amplifying stress. For these reasons, psychological support may help accept the disease and focus on its management and stress management.

Chapter 3: Living with Eczema

Since there is no definitive cure for most eczema, it is necessary to live with them in the best way and manage the present ailments appropriately, thus avoiding relapses. For this reason, it is essential first of all to identify the risk factors and to know how to recognize the reactions of your body since disorders and treatments for eczema can differ significantly from individual to individual. The more you learn to familiarize yourself with eczema, the better you will manage it. A factor that should not be underestimated, often decisive for the quality of life, is the disease's psychological impact. Psycho-physical well-being can be limited by excessive itching that can cause loss of sleep, nervousness, and a sense of inadequacy towards others. In addition to itching, acute skin manifestations, mostly when they occur on the face or other visible parts of the body, can also impact the person's psychological well-being and his everyday social life. In these cases, psychological support is advisable to accept the disease and reduce its skin manifestations. It is also important to talk about your discomfort with other people and point out that it is not a contagious disease.

Prevention

In general, the first real prevention is to keep the skin as healthy as possible and, therefore, defend itself from infections and irritations. This means having constant care of your skin and keeping it hydrated and nourished. Specifically, there is no real prevention of eczema, but some precautions can be followed after its appearance to reduce its disorders and avoid relapses and unwanted effects.

To avoid drying and irritating the skin it is advisable:

- use moisturizing and emollient creams daily
- avoid harsh soaps and shampoos, especially those that contain sodium lauryl sulfate, a foaming agent that tends to cause dryness and irritation
- avoid prolonged showers or baths with very hot water
- dry the skin carefully

- maintain the right degree of humidity in the rooms
- avoid sudden changes in temperature from hot to cold
- prefer cotton fabrics if in direct contact with the skin

In the case of eczema caused by allergies or by contact with irritants, once the responsible substances have been identified, prevention consists in avoiding direct contact with them, in being informed on the names commonly used to indicate them (including synonyms), and on the products that most frequently contain them.

In particular, attention should be paid to:

- body care products, such as perfumes, soaps, shampoos, lotions
- metals that come into contact with the skin, such as buckles, zippers, earrings, bracelets and even cell phones
- substances present in fabrics for clothing and linen (dyes, formaldehyde)
- ingredients found in drugs

It is useful and necessary to learn to read the labels and ingredients of the products to verify the presence, or not, of substances to be avoided.

Diet

Eating certain foods doesn't seem to cause eczema, although it can trigger a flare-up if you already have the condition. Maintaining an eczema-friendly diet is key to overall condition management. Not everyone will have the same reactions or inflammations to the same foods. Below is a list of foods that contain properties that can help reduce eczema flare-ups, but knowing your body and which foods work best for you individually is crucial.

Food to eat

- fatty fish
- apples
- blueberries
- cherries
- broccoli
- spinach
- cabbage
- yogurt
- soy
- dried fruit
- legumes
- oats
- cocoa
- peppers
- oranges
- strawberries
- cauliflower
- pineapple
- mango

Elimination diet

The elimination diet is recommended for people who have been diagnosed with food allergies. If you're unsure what your eczema triggers are, trying the elimination diet may or may not reduce flare-ups. There are many triggers for eczema outside of what you eat, including stress and the environment. This could make it more difficult to determine what's causing your outbreaks. If you wish to try the elimination diet, start by removing specific foods or food groups from what you eat for at least three days to see if your flare-ups subside. For best results, try removing one particular food or food group at a time.

Chapter 4: Breakfast

1) Apple heart biscuits

Ingredients:
- **an egg**
- **100 g of cane sugar**
- **half a bag of yeast**
- **wholemeal flour to taste**
- **a coffee glass of extra virgin olive oil**
- **grated orange peel**

For the apple filling
- **3 apples**
- **2 teaspoons of powdered ginger**
- **the juice of half a lemon**
- **2 tablespoons of brown sugar**

In a bowl, put the egg, brown sugar, grated orange peel, and olive oil. Mix the ingredients with a fork in a circular and continuous pattern until you get a homogeneous and creamy mixture. Stir in the yeast and mix. At this point, add the sifted flour a little at a time, always mixing it with a fork in the bowl. You will see the dough gradually transform, acquire body and shape while remaining soft. For the recipe's success, this is an important step: consider mixing the flour at the rate of a spoon at a time until your liquid and creamy dough become more compact but not hard. Transfer it to a lightly floured pastry board and knead. When it no longer sticks to your hands, your pastry will be ready. Give it a ball shape and place it in the refrigerator for 30 minutes.

Peel and dice the apples, put them in a bowl, add the lemon juice, the ginger powder, and the sugar. Mix well and pour into a non-stick pan. Cook for about 10 minutes (the time varies depending on the quality of the apples chosen) over moderate heat until you get a fragrant and creamy mixture. Leave to cool. Take the pastry, roll it out finely and form circles you will use to shape your cookies. Everything is ready to assemble the ingredients: you will need a bowl with a little water to seal the edges of the biscuits and prevent the contents from escaping: take a pastry base, put the apple filling in the center, with your index finger wet with water moisten the edges of the two pastry bases; then seal the two edges by pressing on them to push the filling towards the center and prevent it from coming out during cooking. With the help of a fork, decorate the edge with light pressure. Repeat until all ingredients are used up. Put the biscuits in a baking tray covered with parchment paper and bake them for 15 minutes at 180 °.

A sprinkle of powdered sugar, and they are ready ... soft, healthy, and very tasty.

2) Savory pie with potatoes and creamy mushrooms

Ingredients:
- **250 g of wholemeal flour**
- **3 tablespoons of sourdough**
- **soya milk**
- **1 teaspoon of brown sugar**
- **2 tablespoons of oil**
- **6 medium potatoes**
- **200 g of mushrooms**
- **100 g of sour cream**
- **150 g of goat cheese**
- **2 cloves of garlic**
- **1 teaspoon of marjoram**
- **2 teaspoons of sweet paprika**
- **sea salt**

Mix the flour with the sourdough, a little salt, and the lukewarm milk necessary to have a firm and homogeneous dough. Knead it for a long time on a table, wrap it into a ball and let it rise in the heat for 4-5 hours. Meanwhile, wash the potatoes and steam them with the peel. While these are getting warm, peel the mushrooms and stew them in a pan with minced garlic, paprika, marjoram, and a little salt. When soft, stir in the cream and crumbled goat cheese. Peel the potatoes and cut them into slices about 1 cm thick.

Roll out two thirds of the dough and use it to line a floured, rectangular, or round, high mold. Spread the potatoes inside, cover with mushrooms. Roll out the rest of the dough so that it covers the entire surface. Seal the edges well, brush with a little warm milk and bake at 180 degrees for 30-35 minutes. Serve the cake hot.

3) Omelette with potatoes and onions

Ingredients:
- **800 g of potatoes**
- **6 eggs**
- **2 onions**
- **2 cloves of garlic**
- **2 tablespoons of oil**
- **1 pinch of nutmeg**
- **1 pinch of parsley**
- **1 pinch of chives**
- **pepper**
- **salt**

Finely slice the onions and garlic. Wash and peel the potatoes and cut them into cubes. Fry the onions and garlic in a pan with olive oil and water, add the potatoes, and cook them until tender. Season with the chopped parsley and chives and mix well. Beat the eggs, add the grated nutmeg to taste, and pour the mixture over the potatoes. When the eggs have hardened, turn the omelette and finish cooking on the other side. Serve immediately.

4)   Buckwheat pancakes in tomato sauce

Ingredients:
- **200 g of buckwheat**
- **1 clove of garlic**
- **salt**
- **½ tablespoon of curry**
- **½ tablespoon of marjoram**
- **½ tablespoon of cumin**
- **breadcrumbs**
- **extra virgin olive oil**

For the sauce
- **1 small onion**
- **400 g of tomato puree**
- **1 bunch of basil**
- **salt and pepper**
- **10 pitted olives**
- **2 tablespoons of oil**

Put the buckwheat in a pot with 500 ml of water, a pinch of salt, and bring to a boil. Cover and cook for 10 minutes, then turn off and let cool with the lid on. Add the spices, garlic, and part of the breadcrumbs; form flattened meatballs, bread them and fry them in boiling oil. Chop and sauté the onion with a little water and oil for about 8-10 minutes; then add the puree, olives, chopped basil, salt, and pepper. Continue cooking for about 30 minutes. Serve the pancakes hot with the sauce.

5)

Tart with pumpkin and walnuts

Ingredients:
- **250 g of flour type 00**
- **50 g of sunflower oil**
- **50 g of rice malt**
- **75 g of soy milk**
- **1 pinch of salt**

For the stuffing:
- **400 g of pumpkin**
- **200 g of shelled and toasted walnuts**
- **100 g of raw cane sugar**
- **1 teaspoon of ground cinnamon**
- **bread crumbs**
- **salt**

Prepare the shortcrust pastry by mixing 250 g of flour, sunflower oil, rice malt, and soy milk. Add a pinch of salt and roll the dough until it is 4-5 mm thick. Roll out the dough into an oiled pan. Aside, stew the peeled pumpkin in a saucepan. Pass it through a vegetable mill and mix in the sugar and cinnamon, adding a few tablespoons of water if necessary. Leave to cool. Spread a sprinkling of breadcrumbs over the dough base and then transfer the pumpkin filling and chopped walnuts. Place in a preheated oven at 180 degrees for 25-30 minutes.

5) Salty muffin

Ingredients:
- **130 g of wholemeal flour**
- **120 g of corn flour**
- **3 teaspoon of curry**
- **1 small carrot**
- **1 piece of leek (the green part)**
- **soya milk**
- **3 tablespoons of oil**
- **1 teaspoon of oregano**
- **3 tablespoon of mixed pumpkin, flax and sunflower seeds**
- **1 sachet of yeast**
- **salt**

Chop the seeds and put them in a bowl. Combine the two flours, curry, oregano, yeast, and salt. Pour in the oil first, then gradually add enough milk to have a soft mixture (about 1 glass). Complete with the diced carrot and the washed and thinly sliced leek. Pour the mixture into a tall, narrow mold lined with baking paper. Bake at 180 degrees for 35-40 minutes. When cooked, allow the muffin to cool, turn it out of the mold and let it cool. Serve with a thick tomato sauce or with chopped and sautéed leeks and carrots.

6) Lentil crepes

Ingredients:
- **100-120 of cooked and well dried lentils**
- **3 tablespoons of flour**
- **100-120 ml of oat milk**
- **2 teaspoons of turmeric**
- **salt and black pepper**
- **oil**

For the filling:
- **tomato sauce**

Mix the cooled lentils with turmeric, a little salt, and black pepper. Dilute the flour in the vegetable milk. Add salt and gradually pour the mixture over the lentils. Mix well. Heat a small non-stick pan with a thin layer of oil and pour half of the dough at a time. Cook each crepe on both sides for a few minutes until it is golden brown. Serve the pancakes hot, sprinkled with a drizzle of oil.

7) Coconut biscuits

Ingredients:
- •300 g of flour
- •100 g of butter
- 120 g of brown sugar
- •50 g of ground coconut
- •1 small egg
- •milk
- •1 heaped teaspoon of ground cinnamon
- •2 ground cloves
- •1 teaspoon of ground ginger
- •1 pinch of salt

Put the sugar in the mixer and operate to make it fine and homogeneous. Let the butter soften at room temperature. Work the two ingredients with a whisk until they are well blended, then add the coconut and the beaten egg. Gradually add the flour previously sifted and mixed with the salt and spices. If needed, wet with a little milk to have a firm and homogeneous mixture. Shape into a ball and let it rest for 60 minutes in a cool place. Roll out the dough that is not too thin and make the biscuits with the appropriate molds. Brush them with a little milk and arrange them on a baking sheet lined with baking paper. Cook them at 200 ° for about 12 minutes, turning them once. They must not overcook; otherwise, they harden; remove them still a little tender. Transfer them to a wire rack to cool and store them in a tin box. After a few days, they are even better.

8) Date and almond cake

Ingredients:
- **230 g of flour 0**
- **40 g of corn malt**
- **40 ml of corn oil**
- **5 g of fresh brewer's yeast**
- **1 small teaspoon of vanilla powder**
- **the grated peel of 1/2 lemon**
- **60 ml of warm water**

For the date cream
- **500 g of pitted dates**
- **350 ml of water**
- **1 pinch of salt**

To decorate
mixture of malt and hot water in a ratio of 3 to 1
- **20 g of flaked almonds**

Wash the dates and cook covered and over low heat with water and a pinch of salt until the cooking liquid is completely absorbed. Blend and let the cream cool. Proceed by preparing the cake dough: melt the brewer's yeast in warm water and leave it aside. In the meantime, take a large bowl to put the flour, a pinch of salt, vanilla, and lemon peel. Make a hole in the center and stir in the corn oil and then, little by little, the yeast and malt. Then work the dough by combining all the ingredients, always with more energy, and helping yourself with a bit of flour until you have a ball free of lumps. Flour a work surface and transfer the dough into it: knead it for about 5 minutes, with continuous and circular movements, until it is elastic and smooth. Let it rest for 30 minutes. With a rolling pin, make a sheet by pressing the dough, starting from the center and proceeding outwards. When you have obtained a disk of about 30 cm, place it on a baking sheet lined with parchment paper, and with your thumbs, press the internal corners of the pastry well, shaping the edge. Spread the date cream on the base and cook in a preheated oven at 200 ° for 40 minutes. Once out of the oven, brush the cake's surface with the polish and decorate with a cascade of briefly toasted almond flakes in a non-stick pan.

9) Kamut flour biscuits

Ingredients:
- **250 g of kamut flour**
- **150 g of maple syrup**
- **50 g of chopped and toasted almonds**
- **70 ml of corn oil**
- **50 g of raisins**
- **50 g of unsweetened cocoa powder**
- **20 g of yeast**
- **200 ml of warm water**
- **1 teaspoon of vanilla**
- **the grated peel of ½ orange**
- **1 pinch of salt**

In a bowl, combine the oil and maple syrup, mixing well. Gather the dry ingredients in a bowl: the flour, the chopped almonds, the unsweetened cocoa, the baking powder, the salt, and the vanilla, mix them evenly and add the raisins, water, and the mixture with the syrup. 'Maple. Work with your hands until you get a soft and smooth dough: lifting a bit of the dough with one hand and letting it fall slowly. Pour some of the dough into the pastry bag and squeeze to form corrugated discs on the pan (space the cookies apart, so they have room to rise). Bake the cookies in the oven at 200 ° for 20 minutes. Let them cool and serve them.

10) Apple and walnut muffins

Ingredients:
- **125 g of flour 0**
- **40 g of walnut kernels**
- **30 g of small rolled oats**
- **150 ml of milk**
- **90 ml of honey**
- **1 apple**
- **1 egg**
- **30 ml of peanut oil**
- **8 g vanilla baking powder (1/2 sachet)**

Start preparing the apple and walnut muffins by placing the oat flakes with milk in a bowl and letting them rest for 15 minutes. After this time, add the honey, the egg and mix with a hand whisk. Add the oil, the chopped walnuts, the peeled and diced apple, and complete with the sifted flour together with the baking powder. Stir again with a spatula to mix all the ingredients well. Transfer the dough into the special pan with muffin molds, greased and floured, sprinkle each with some oat flakes on the surface, and bake them in the oven for 25-30 minutes. Let the apple and nut muffins rest for 5-10 minutes, then remove them from the molds and let them cool on a wire rack.

11) Orange Plumcake

Ingredients:
- 2 eggs at room temperature
- 170 g of granulated sugar
- 160 ml of orange juice
- 80 ml of seed oil
- 210 g of flour 00
- 50 g of potato starch
- 16 g of baking powder for cakes
- 1 pinch of cinnamon
- 2 organic blood oranges

Start preparing the orange plum cake by whipping the eggs with sugar and cinnamon in the planetary mixer or a large bowl until you get a frothy mixture. Add the finely grated zest of 1 orange and mix. Then add the seed oil and the orange juice, filtered through a colander, taking care to incorporate them well. Continue with the sifted flour together with the starch and baking powder. Pour half of the mixture into a 25x11 cm loaf pan. Place 4 or 5 thinly sliced orange halves on top, cover with the remaining mixture, and spread other orange slices in half on the surface. Transfer to a preheated oven at 180 degrees for about 45 minutes. At the end of cooking, do the classic "toothpick test" to make sure that the cake is ready. Remove the orange plum cake from the oven and let it cool completely before turning it out of the mold and serving.

12) Light pancake

Ingredients:
- 100 g of egg whites
- 125 g of Greek yogurt
- 80 g of wholemeal flour
- 2 tablespoons of honey
- 2 tablespoons of skim milk
- 1 tablespoon of seed oil
- 1 teaspoon of baking powder for cakes
- 1/4 teaspoon of baking soda
- 1/2 vanilla bean

TO SERVE
- honey
- blueberries or other fruit to taste

To make the light pancakes, first, collect the egg whites in a bowl. Beat them with a hand whisk for 30 seconds. Add the Greek yogurt, vanilla seeds, honey, and oil. Work everything until you get a homogeneous cream. Add the wholemeal flour, sifted with baking powder and baking soda, and mix it by slowly adding the milk. You will need to obtain a smooth and homogeneous batter with a slightly thick but not too thick consistency. Grease a non-stick pan with the seed oil and heat it well, removing the excess oil with kitchen paper. Pour a ladle of batter and let it spread out into a disc. When you notice large bubbles appear on the surface, turn the pancake and continue cooking on the other side. When cooked, transfer to a plate. Proceed in this way until the batter is used up. Serve the light pancakes warm with honey and blueberries.

13) Blueberry butter-free donut

Ingredients:
- **2 eggs at room temperature**
- **100 g of granulated sugar**
- **100 g of light brown sugar**
- **100 g of plain yogurt**
- **75 g of seed oil**
- **200 g of flour 00**
- **1/2 vanilla bean**
- **10 g of baking powder**
- **1 basket of blueberries**
- **a pinch of salt**
- **powdered sugar**

To make the blueberry butter-free donut, start whipping the eggs together with the sugar, a pinch of salt, and the vanilla seeds (extracted from the berry by cutting it lengthwise and scratching it with a small knife). Whip until the mixture is light and fluffy. Then add the yogurt and oil, mixing with a hand whisk to incorporate them perfectly. Then add the flour, sieved with baking powder, and mix well. Finally, stir in the blueberries, stirring gently so as not to break them. Pour the dough into a donut mold, with a diameter of 18 cm, previously greased and floured. Transfer to the oven, preheated to 180 °, for about 45 minutes or in any case until by inserting a toothpick into the cake it comes out dry. Remove the cake from the oven and let it cool before turning it out. Sprinkle the blueberry butter-free donut with powdered sugar to taste before serving.

14) Gluten-free pancakes

Ingredients:
- 220 g of soy milk
- 1 tsp apple cider vinegar
- 15 g of seed oil
- 1/4 vanilla bean or 1 teaspoon vanilla extract (optional)
- 80 g of buckwheat flour
- 40 g of rice flour
- 25 g of corn starch or potato starch
- 4 g of baking powder
- 15 g of whole cane sugar
- a pinch of salt
- oil to oil the pan

TO SERVE
- Maple syrup
- raspberries or other fresh fruit to taste

To prepare gluten-free pancakes in a bowl, combine the soy milk, vinegar, seed oil, and vanilla. Stir and let it rest. Separately, sift the flours with the starch and yeast. Add the sugar and a pinch of salt. Mix the flours with a whisk, and then pour the liquid mixture. Stir vigorously until the dough is smooth and without lumps. Heat a non-stick pan over medium-high heat and cover the surface with a few drops of oil. When the pan is hot, pour 2 tablespoons of mixture for each pancake. When bubbles form on the surface, and the edges darken, flip the pancakes and cook the other side. Repeat the process until the dough is used up, ensuring that the pan does not get too hot. If so, remove the pan from the heat for a minute. Serve the gluten-free pancakes hot with 2-3 teaspoons of maple syrup and fresh fruit to taste.

15) Good morning sandwiches

Ingredients:
- 75 g brown rice flour
- 100 g flour 0
- 150 g corn starch
- 38 g potato starch
- 36 g coconut powder
- 4 g xanthan gum
- 15 g granulated sugar
- 8 g salt
- 15 g brewer's yeast
- 270 g whole eggs
- 200 g coconut drink
- 60 g cocoa butter
- 50 g sunflower oil

FOR THE GASKET
- 50 g oil seeds (flax, chia, green pumpkin, sunflower)
- 150 g dried fruit (figs, apricots, plums, cranberries)
- 100 g cereal flakes (rice, corn, buckwheat)

In the planetary mixer with leaf, pre-mix all the powders, including salt and sugar; increasing the speed, gradually add the crumbled brewer's yeast. Combine the whole eggs and the coconut drink until the dough is smooth and soft. Melt the cocoa butter with the oil and add it to the mixture a little at a time. Finally, add the rehydrated oil seeds with half the weight of water. Portion the mixture obtained into the molds. Garnish with partially rehydrated dried fruit, cover with a layer of flakes, also rehydrated with a little water, and let rise covered with nylon cloth for food at 26-28 ° C for 60-90 '. Bake in the oven at 170 ° C for 10-15 minutes until fully developed and opening to complete cooking.

Chapter 5: Snacks, appetizers and side dishes

1) Sauteed spinach with dried fruit

Ingredients:
- 500 g of spinach
- 50 g of dried apples
- 50 g of raisins
- a little pine nuts
- 1 clove of garlic
- extra virgin olive oil as needed
- Salt to taste.

Soak the apples and raisins for about 20 minutes in warm water. Clean and wash the spinach. Blanch them in lightly salted water for a few minutes. Drain them by squeezing them well, and cut them coarsely. Fry the garlic in a pan greased with oil, add the spinach, and after a while, the raisins and well-squeezed apples, pine nuts, and salt. Let it cook over high heat for a few minutes, season with salt, and serve the spinach hot.

2) Carrot puree with green olives

Ingredients:
- **500 g of carrots**
- **1 teaspoon of paprika**
- **2 teaspoons of cumin**
- **3 tablespoons of rice vinegar**
- **2 minced garlic cloves**
- **1 tablespoon of oil**
- **grated ginger juice**
- **green olives for garnish**
- **salt and pepper**

Peel and cut the carrots into rings and place them in a steamer basket. Cook them, covered, in a saucepan with lightly salted boiling water. After about ten minutes, check that they are soft. Blend them with the rest of the ingredients and a little cooking water to obtain a puree's consistency. Let the puree rest for a couple of hours so that the flavors blend. If you prefer, put it in the fridge for a while. Serve at room temperature or slightly chilled.

3) Eggplant and tofu meatballs

Ingredients:
- **100 g of tofu**
- **1 large eggplant**
- **1 clove of garlic**
- **2 sprigs of parsley**
- **1 tablespoon of flour**
- **4 tablespoons of breadcrumbs**
- **salt**
- **oil to taste**

Cook the whole eggplant in the oven; once cooked, sauté its pulp in a pan in a garlic sauce. Season with salt and add the crumbled tofu. Mix the ingredients, if necessary, with a little flour. Complete the preparation with chopped parsley. Prepare meatballs the size of an apricot, dip them in breadcrumbs, bake them or fry them in a pan, according to preference.

4) Turmeric chickpeas sauteed with radicchio, dates and almonds

Ingredients:
- 1 head of red radicchio
- 400 g of cooked chickpeas
- 1 clove of garlic
- 1 tablespoon of turmeric powder
- extra virgin olive oil
- ½ teaspoon of cumin powder
- 7-8 pitted dates
- 1 handful of shelled almonds
- sea salt

In a heavy-bottomed pan, heat a little oil and brown the peeled and chopped garlic. Add the chickpeas, let them flavor, and add turmeric and cumin, stir, and lightly salt. Cook over high heat for about a minute, stirring constantly. Add the peeled and cleaned radicchio; it must wither for a couple of minutes. Just before removing from the heat, add the dates cut into small pieces. Complete with the chopped almonds, a drizzle of extra virgin olive oil, and bring to the table.

5)   Rice and zucchini croquettes with saffron sauce

Ingredients:
For the croquettes:
- **350 g of brown rice**
- **850 ml of water**
- **800 g of zucchini**
- **2 tablespoons of oil**
- **1 teaspoon of salt**
- **1 bunch of parsley**
- **1 clove of garlic**
- **salt and pepper**

For the saffron sauce:
- **250 ml of soy milk**
- **30 ml of oil**
- **30 g of rice flour**
- **1 sachet of saffron and salt**

Sauté the chopped garlic and parsley in a little oil. Add and stew the sliced zucchini with salt and pepper for 10 minutes. Puree about 1/3 of the zucchini. Wash the rice, drain it and cook it in salted water, covered and without stirring, for about 35 minutes. Season the rice with the salt and the zucchini not passed, stir and continue cooking for another 5 minutes. Let it cool (if it is too soft, let it cool completely or add some breadcrumbs), then form some meatballs that you will bake in the oven at 200 ° for about 15-20 minutes. To prepare the sauce, brown the flour in a saucepan with the oil, then add the milk. Bring to a boil and let it thicken over low heat, stirring with a whisk. Salt and add the saffron and the zucchini puree.

6) Carrot and sweet potato roll with millet

Ingredients:
- **200 g of carrots**
- **1 sweet potato**
- **1 tablespoon of corn starch**
- **200 g of cooked millet**
- **3 tablespoons of oil**
- **salt**

To garnish
- **100 g of peeled pumpkin**
- **a few leaves of salad**
- **1 tablespoon of oil**
- **salt**

Clean the carrots and the potato, chop them and steam them for about 10 minutes. Let them cool, then blend them in the mixer with the millet, starch, oil, and salt. Remove the salami mixture and wrap it in cotton gauze, closing them like candy with a piece of string. Steam them for 15-20 minutes. Wait until they are completely cold and cut them into slices. Wash the salad, dry it and cut it into strips; coarsely grate the pumpkin. Arrange the rolls on a serving dish, surround them with the prepared garnish seasoned with oil and salt.

7) Rice balls with broccoli and almond pesto

Ingredients:
For the stuffing
• **leftover already seasoned rice, or other cereal. If you use leftover rice, millet, amaranth and quinoa, the recipe is also suitable for celiacs.**
• **extra virgin olive oil or seeds for frying**

For the batter
• **chickpea flour**
• **water q.s.**
• **a pinch of salt**
• **breadcrumbs**

For the broccoli and almond pesto
• **half a fresh broccoli**
• **80 g of almonds**
• **the juice of half a lemon**
• **a clove of garlic**
• **a large tuft of fresh parsley**
• **Salt to taste.**
• **extra virgin olive oil as needed**

Cut your broccoli into small pieces and steam it or cook it in a pot in hot water for a maximum of 10 minutes. Put it in the blender and add the remaining ingredients: the garlic clove into small pieces, the parsley, the lemon juice, the almonds, the salt, and the olive oil. Blend vigorously, help yourself using a little water if necessary (the one used for cooking broccoli, for example), taste, and season with salt. Put the pesto in a large bowl and let the ingredients rest.

At this point, we proceed with the preparation and cooking of the meatballs. In a bowl, mix the chickpea flour with water, avoiding the formation of lumps. Mix vigorously until you get a thick and homogeneous batter. Add a pinch of salt. Prepare a dish with the center's breadcrumbs: you can make your breading even tastier by adding chopped aromatic herbs, garlic or onion, sesame seeds, or chopped hazelnuts. With wet hands, take some leftover rice and form a ball to dip into the batter first and then pass it into the breadcrumbs. Repeat the operation until the dough is used up.

Prepare a pot with a high bottom and put the oil to heat. Once the temperature is reached, start frying your meatballs for a few minutes until they are golden, and place them in a dish lined with absorbent paper. Take a serving dish, place your hot and crunchy meatballs in the center, bring to the table and serve them accompanied by the broccoli and almond pesto sauce. Delicious!

8)   Fennel in orange cream

Ingredients:
- **2 medium fennel**
- **1 cup of cashews**
- **125 ml of orange juice**
- **2 teaspoons of dried mint**
- **1 pinch of chilli**
- **1 tablespoon of oil**
- **½ teaspoon of salt**
- **1 teaspoon of agave syrup**

Wash the fennel, cut them into four parts, and, using a mandolin, slice them finely. Sprinkle it with salt and let it rest. Meanwhile, prepare the cream. Put the cashews in the blender with the orange juice, mint, chili pepper, oil, salt, and agave syrup and mix until the mixture is fluid and without lumps. Drain the fennel water and season with the cream.

9)   Rice and seitan croquettes

Ingredients:
- **200 g of brown rice**
- **100 g of seitan**
- **1 onion**
- **1 carrot**
- **2 teaspoons of fresh grated ginger**
- **bread crumbs**
- **oil and salt to taste**

Beat the vegetables and add the grated ginger. Brown in a saucepan and cover. Chop the seitan, which will be added to the vegetables when they are already wilted. Meanwhile, boil the rice separately with enough water for its cooking. When cooked, add it to the vegetables and mix it for a few minutes before turning off the heat. Leave to cool. Then obtain some balls to pass in the breadcrumbs and place on a pan brushed with oil. Brown the croquettes in the oven for about twenty minutes at about 200 ° C.

10) Pizza with buckwheat flour and rice flour

Ingredients:
- 300 g of rice flour
- 100 g of buckwheat flour
- 1 sachet of yeast
- 1 handful of salt
- 3 tablespoons of oil

For the filling
- 200 g of tomato puree
- 250 g of blanched tofu
- 400 g of zucchini
- 1 clove of garlic
- 1 artichoke
- stoned olives
- salt and oil
- oregano or basil

Cut the zucchini into slices and sauté them in a pan with oil, minced garlic, salt, and olives for about 10 minutes; they must be al dente. Gather the sifted flours, salt, and yeast in a bowl. Add a tablespoon of oil, about 260 ml of water, and knead until you get a rather soft dough. Spread it with your hands on a greased pizza pan (or better still, lined with baking paper), which you will completely cover with the sauce seasoned with oil and salt. Bake in a preheated oven for about 15 minutes at 190 °. Remove from the oven and spread on the surface the tofu chopped with your hands, the zucchini, oregano, and artichoke, peeled and finely sliced. Return to the oven for another 10-15 minutes at 170 °. Serve with the rest of the raw oil.

11) Red cabbage with spices

Ingredients:
- ½ red cabbage
- 3 apples
- 1 orange
- 3 tablespoons of raisins
- 3 tablespoons of pine nuts
- ½ glass of apple vinegar
- 2 tablespoons of oil
- 2 cloves
- cinnamon powder
- nutmeg
- salt

Cut the cabbage into thin strips and toss it in a heavy-bottomed pot with oil until it "sweats." Add the orange juice, the thinly sliced peel, and the apple vinegar. Lower the heat and add the apples cut into small pieces, the cloves, the previously soaked raisins, and a nice pinch of salt to the pot. Mix well, cover, and cook for about 40 minutes or until the cabbage is very soft. During the last 10 minutes of cooking, add the spices and pine nuts. It is even better to eat the next day.

12) Brussels sprouts with chestnuts and currants

Ingredients:
- **350 g of Brussels sprouts**
- **12-15 boiled chestnuts**
- **2-3 sprigs of red currant**
- **1 clove of garlic**
- **oil**
- **salt**
- **pepper**
- **a few sprigs of thyme**
- **a few drops of balsamic vinegar**

Cook the sprouts in lightly salted boiling water for a few minutes, until tender; drain well and pour into a pan where the oil has been flavored with the crushed garlic. Brown briefly, then add the chestnuts and mix again. Season with pepper, thyme, and a few drops of balsamic vinegar. Garnish with the currants and serve immediately.

13) Potato and cauliflower patties with yogurt sauce

Ingredients:
- **300 ml of soy yogurt**
- **250 g of cauliflower**
- **450 g of potatoes**
- **150 g of chickpea flour**
- **1 tablespoon of chopped fresh parsley**
- **1 teaspoon of turmeric**
- **1 teaspoon of thyme**
- **oil**
- **salt and pepper**

Clean the cauliflower, divide it into florets and wash it. Peel the potatoes, rinse them, and cut them into squares. Steam the two ingredients for about 15 minutes. While they are cooking, mix the yogurt with a pinch of salt and parsley. Set it aside. Let the vegetables cool and mash them with a potato masher, collecting the past in a bowl. Add the chickpea flour, thyme, turmeric, salt, and pepper. Stir with the spoon. When the mixture is homogeneous (if it were too soft, add more chickpea flour), take small portions with wet hands and make spherical balls with a diameter of about 4 cm. Arrange them in a pan brushed with oil. Bake at 180 degrees for 15 minutes, turning them a couple of times. Serve hot, accompanied with the yogurt sauce.

14) Mashed fava beans

Ingredients:

- **250 g of broad beans**

- **1 white onion**

- **4 tablespoons of oil**

- **2 cloves of garlic**

- **salt**

Rinse the previously soaked broad beans overnight and boil them with the garlic for about 2 hours in a saucepan. Peel and chop the onion; put them in a large pan with a tablespoon of oil and a glass of water. Salt and cook over medium heat, uncovered, for about 10 minutes, until the liquid is used up. In the end, turn off and season with a little oil. Blend the beans and onion by immersion, season with the salt and the remaining oil; serve as a side dish.

15) Baked zucchini with curry, pumpkin seeds and chia

Ingredients:
- 5 zucchini
- 4 tablespoons of pumpkin seeds
- 1 tablespoon of chia seeds
- 1 teaspoon of curry powder
- lemon juice
- freshly ground black pepper
- extra virgin olive oil
- sea salt

Wash the zucchini well and cut them into 4 lengthwise. Put them in a ceramic pan, sprinkle them with oil, salt them and bake them at 180 °. Cook them for about 25 minutes, turning them often. Let the vegetables cool slightly. Season with lemon juice, more oil if necessary, season with salt, pepper and complete with pumpkin and chia seeds, which you will distribute on the surface with the curry. Serve immediately.

Chapter 6: Single course

1) Radicchio and pear risotto with spices

Ingredients:
- **320 g of brown rice**
- **250 g of radicchio**
- **200 g of pears**
- **a few walnut kernels**
- **oil**
- **1 l of vegetable broth**
- **½ glass of white wine**
- **3 cloves**
- **the juice of ½ lemon**
- **salt**

Cut the pears into cubes and sprinkle them with lemon so that they do not darken. Reduce the radicchio (except four or five leaves) into thin strips. Sauté the radicchio with the cloves in a saucepan with some olive oil for a few minutes, add the pears and cook for another minute. Transfer everything to a bowl. Clean the pan's cooking bottom, pour a couple of tablespoons of oil, and toast the washed and drained rice. Deglaze with the wine, season over high heat for one minute. Add the boiling broth a little at a time, waiting for it to be absorbed before adding more. Halfway through cooking, add the radicchio and cooked pears; season with salt. Serve the risotto in the wave, and garnish it with the walnut kernels and raw radicchio leaves.

2) Pumpkin rice

Ingredients:
- **1 cup of brown rice**
- **1 onion**
- **400 g of clean pumpkin**
- **3 cups of vegetable broth**
- **1 sprig of rosemary**
- **3 tablespoons of oil**

Put the rice in a saucepan with 2 cups of broth. Cover and bring it to a boil, then lower the heat and cook slowly for an hour. Meanwhile, finely chop the onion and transfer it to a pan just covered with broth. Let it soften over medium heat for a few minutes before adding the diced pumpkin and rosemary leaves. Pour in the remaining broth and cook over low heat for 10-15 minutes. Add the pumpkin to the cooked rice and leave to rest for 5 minutes. Season with oil and salt, stir, and serve.

3) Mushroom flan

Ingredients:
- **300 g of potatoes**
- **100 g of mushrooms**
- **100 g of leeks**
- **1 egg**
- **1 teaspoon of cinnamon**
- **100 g of tofu**
- **60 ml of soy milk**
- **1 tablespoon of oil**
- **1 tablespoon of water**
- **Salt and Pepper To Taste**

Wash the potatoes and steam them with the peel. When they are soft, pass them with a potato masher in a bowl. Add the egg, milk, and cinnamon. Meanwhile, peel the leeks, wash them and slice them finely. Let them dry in a pan with oil and water. Add the cleaned mushrooms and cut them into slices. Cook over high heat to evaporate the mushroom vegetation water. At this point, add the tofu, salt, and pepper. Line a rectangular mold with high sides with baking paper. Spread half of the mashed potatoes on top, cover with the mushrooms, and finish with the rest of the mash. Bake for about 10 minutes in an oven heated to 200 ° C. Let the flan cool and serve cut into slices.

4)   Quinoa with roasted carrots

Ingredients:
- **250 g of quinoa**
- **4-5 carrots**
- **4 shallots**
- **1/2 tablespoon of cumin**
- **1/2 tablespoon of turmeric**
- **1 handful of toasted pine nuts**
- **1 handful of parsley and very finely chopped celery**
- **extra virgin olive oil**
- **salt and pepper**

Peel the shallots and halve them; cut the carrots in four lengthwise and then into chunks. Put the vegetables in a pan seasoned with oil, cumin, and salt. Bake at 180 degrees for about 30 minutes, turning them now and then until they are well roasted. Meanwhile, wash the quinoa well in cold water, drain it in a tightly meshed colander and rinse again; drain well and dry briefly in a pan with two tablespoons of oil, turmeric, and pepper. Pour in boiling water equal to twice the quinoa's volume, add salt, cover, and cook on a very low flame for 15-20 minutes until the liquid is completely absorbed. Shell the quinoa well and mix it with the vegetables, also collecting their cooking juices with the pine nuts, celery, and parsley. Serve immediately.

<h3 align="center">5)   Chickpea flans with black cabbage</h3>

Ingredients:
- **400 g of boiled and drained chickpeas**
- **500 g of black cabbage**
- **2 cloves of garlic**
- **vegetable broth**
- **2 tablespoons of lemon juice**
- **100 g of sunflower seeds**
- **60-80 g of breadcrumbs**
- **1 teaspoon of thyme**
- **salt**
- **3 tablespoons of oil**

Remove the black cabbage from the rib, wash it, and put it in a saucepan with the minced garlic. Add salt and thyme. Cook over medium heat for about ten minutes, adding a little broth when needed. In the end, let it cool and go to the mixer. Transfer the vegetables to a plate. Collect the drained chickpeas, lemon juice, sunflower seeds, and salt in a blender. Finely chop them with the help of a little broth. Pour everything into a bowl with three quarters of the black cabbage. Add the breadcrumbs necessary to have a compact but still soft mixture. Grease 4 molds of the desired shape with a little oil. Bake at 190 degrees for 15-20 minutes. Serve the flans directly in the molds, accompanied by the cabbage, and seasoned with the remaining oil.

6)   Cous cous with cabbage and pumpkin

Ingredients:
- **250 g of couscous**
- **200 ml of hot water**
- **2 slices of pumpkin**
- **half cabbage**
- **half a savoy cabbage**
- **a shallot**
- **10-12 dried tomatoes**
- **the grated rind of a lemon**
- **extra virgin olive oil as needed**
- **half a small pepper**
- **Salt to taste.**
- **a sprig of fresh parsley**

To cook the couscous: bring 200 ml of water to a boil in a saucepan. Meanwhile, in a large pan, lightly toast the couscous, stirring for a few minutes. Then add two tablespoons of oil and mix well. As soon as the water boils, add a pinch of salt, pour in the couscous, mix with a fork, turn off the heat and cover tightly with a lid for 5 minutes. At this point, you can open and shell your couscous with the help of your hands, which will be well cooked and separated. Leave it in the pot with the lid on and dedicate yourself to preparing the vegetables. Wash the savoy cabbage, and cabbage leaves well and cut them into strips. Clean the pumpkin (you can decide whether to eat it with the peel) and cut it into cubes. Take the dried tomatoes and cut them into small pieces. Put all these ingredients in a bowl. In a saucepan, heat a little water that can be used for cooking the vegetables; alternatively, you can use vegetable broth. In a large pan, heat two tablespoons of extra virgin olive oil with half a small chili pepper. Sauté briefly and stir in the vegetables. Mix well and add a little hot water to cook the vegetables, which must remain crunchy and tasty. Cover with a lid and, often stirring and incorporating water or broth if necessary, cook for 10-15 minutes maximum. Just before turning off the heat, add salt and grate the peel of half a lemon. Then take your couscous, knead it briefly with your hands and add it to the wok or pan with the vegetable sauce. Stir vigorously and serve hot, garnishing each dish with a sprinkle of fresh parsley. It is a simple and inexpensive dish, with beautiful colors that make it very tasty even for children.

7) Broccoli and sweet potato pie

Ingredients:
- **300 g of sweet potatoes**
- **400 g of broccoli**
- **2 cloves of garlic**
- **1 bunch of parsley**
- **1 glass of vegetable broth**
- **3 tablespoons of oil**
- **salt**

Peel and wash the sweet potatoes, then cut them into slices that are not too thick. Peel and clean the broccoli; slice the stems and divide the flowers into florets. Finely chop garlic and parsley. Line a baking sheet with parchment paper and brush it with a tablespoon of oil mixed with water. Make the first layer with the potatoes and a pinch of salt, a second with the broccoli and a little more salt, a third with garlic and parsley. Finish with the potatoes and pour over all the broth. Bake at 190 degrees for about 40 minutes. When cooked, season with the remaining oil and serve.

8) Green rolls

Ingredients:
- **a few leaves of Chinese cabbage (or savoy cabbage)**
- **1 bunch of chard**
- **natural sauerkraut**

Bring plenty of water to a boil, add a pinch of salt and the whole cabbage leaves; cook them until tender and let them drain. Cook the chard in the same water, leaving the leaves whole but separated from the stems, which must cook a little longer. They must maintain a bright green color. Drain them well, squeezing away the excess water. Then wrap the chard, and a sprig of sauerkraut in the cabbage leaves to make rolls. Cut each roll into two pieces.

9) Barley flans with beetroot sauce

Ingredients:
- 350 g of pearl barley
- 850 ml of water
- 2 large eggplants:
- 300 g of zucchini
- 250 g of fresh tofu
- 50 g of sunflower seeds
- 3 clean cloves of garlic
- 3 tablespoons of oil
- 1 lemon (juice)
- 1 teaspoon of sweet paprika
- 1 teaspoon of cumin
- 1 bunch of clean basil
- salt
- pepper

For the beetroot sauce
- 500 g of red beets
- 50 g of pitted black olives
- 100-200 ml of soy milk
- 3 tablespoons of sunflower oil
- 1 tablespoon of lemon juice

Wash the barley, drain it, and put it in a saucepan with salted water. Bring to a boil and reduce to low if necessary with the flame spreader. Cover and cook without stirring for about 35 minutes. Drain the peeled and diced eggplants. Wash and cut the zucchini into slices. Chop the garlic and basil. Mix the lemon juice and paprika. Fry the mixture with cumin, diced tofu, and salt in oil for 3 minutes. Add the squeezed eggplants and brown them for 5 minutes, stirring several times. Add the zucchini and ½ cup of water and cook for 8-10 minutes over medium heat; finally, add the salt and pepper and cook for 2 minutes.

Toast the sunflower seeds for 15 minutes in a preheated oven at 170 °. When the barley is cooked, season it with eggplants and tofu, put the lid on, and continue cooking for 5 minutes. Oil the molds and fill them with pressing them well with a spoon; let them rest for a few minutes. For the sauce, wash the beets and boil them in lightly salted water, drain, let them cool and peel them. Then cut them into small pieces and blend them with the black olives, sunflower oil, lemon juice. Finally, add the soy milk a little at a time until it forms a smooth and creamy sauce. Turn the flans over onto serving plates, cover with a couple of tablespoons of sauce and serve.

10) Stuffed peppers

Ingredients:
- **4 red peppers**
- **1 tablespoon of sour cream**
- **vegetable broth**
- **2 spring onions with the green part**
- **1 bunch of parsley**
- **1 teaspoon of dill**
- **1 teaspoon of paprika**
- **1 clove of garlic**
- **salt and chilli**

Halve the peppers lengthwise and remove the core and white ribs. Wash and dry them. Bake them for 15 minutes to make them soften a little. Meanwhile, chop the cheese and put it in a blender with the sliced garlic, the cleaned parsley, the dill, the paprika, and the chili. Add the peeled and shredded onions and the sour cream. Blend everything with the help of the broth necessary to have a homogeneous and not too soft mixture. Stuff the half peppers and bake again for about 10 minutes. Serve the dish warm or hot.

11) Indian rice

Ingredients:
- **300 g of wholemeal basmati rice**
- **1 carrot**
- **200 g of peas**
- **2 shallots**
- **1 piece of cinnamon**
- **2 cardamom capsules**
- **1 heaped teaspoon of turmeric**
- **1 clove**
- **1 bay leaf**
- **1 tablespoon of raisins**
- **20 almonds**
- **3 tablespoons of oil**
- **salt and pepper**

Put the rice in a saucepan, cover it with 800 ml of water, close with the lid, and boil. Turn down the heat. Rinse the raisins and soak them in warm water for about ten minutes. Put the chopped shallots in a pan with the cinnamon, the cardamom seeds, the turmeric, the clove, and the bay leaf. Add the soaking water from the raisins and let it soften over medium heat, stirring often. Transfer to the saucepan with the rice. When 30 minutes have passed, add the peas, raisins, and carrot cut into cubes. Cook for another 15-20 minutes until the liquid has run out. Remove the bay leaf, the carnation, and the cinnamon. Season with salt, season with oil and pepper. Complete with the sliced almonds and serve.

12) Spelled and leek lasagna

Ingredients:
- **300 g of lasagne**
- **2 leeks**
- **250 g of mozzarella**
- **70 g of parmesan cheese**
- **extra virgin olive oil**
- **½ glass of milk**

Clean the leeks, cut them lengthwise, and soak them in freshwater for about 30 minutes. Meanwhile, in a full pot of boiling water, cook the lasagna for about 5 minutes and set it aside. Drain the leeks and put them to stew in a pan with a drizzle of oil without adding salt because they are already delicious. Cook them for about twenty minutes. Take a pan, preferably rectangular, and form the layers: start by placing a layer of pasta on the pan's bottom and lay the leeks on top. Take the mozzarella, cut it into small pieces, and put them on top of the leeks. Finish with a sprinkling of parmesan cheese. Continue to alternate puff pastry, leek, mozzarella, and parmesan, until all the ingredients are used up. Once the last sheet is finished, pour the milk over the lasagna and complete it with a shower of parmesan cheese. Bake for 25 minutes at 180 °.

13) Spaghetti in tofu cream with spinach and hazelnuts

Ingredients:
- **350 g of wholemeal spaghetti**
- **200 g of fresh spinach**
- **80 g of hazelnuts**

For the olive tofu cream
- **200 g of natural tofu**
- **the juice of half a lemon**
- **1 cup of capers**
- **1 cup of olives**
- **a large tuft of chopped parsley**
- **3 tablespoons of olive oil**
- **a tablespoon of soy sauce**
- **a pinch of salt**
- **1 small clove of garlic**

Put the water on the fire to cook the pasta; once it reaches a boil, add salt and throw the wholemeal spaghetti. In the meantime, take a saucepan with a little water and put it on the stove: as soon as it boils, add a pinch of salt and dip the natural tofu block cut into small pieces. Boil for a minute, drain, and put it in the blender, where you will add the olives without the stones, the sprig of parsley, the capers, the juice of half a lemon, the clove of garlic, the oil, the soy sauce, and the pinch of salt. To soften, you can add a few tablespoons of the tofu boiling water. Blend until you get a soft and homogeneous cream that you will keep aside. Then wash the fresh spinach leaves; you can roughly cut them or leave them whole. Dry them and keep them aside. Then take a non-stick pan and toast the hazelnuts, coarsely chopped. Drain the pasta and put it in a large bowl, and add the tofu cream to the olives; if necessary, help yourself with a little tofu cooking water, as above. Add the fresh spinach leaves, toasted hazelnuts, and finally a drizzle of raw oil. If you wish, you can also add a splash of fresh oregano or paprika powder. Serve the spaghetti hot and steaming. Simple and tasty!

14) Pasta with broccoli

Ingredients:
- **400 g of pasta**
- **1 large broccoli**
- **1 clove of garlic**
- **4 tablespoons of chopped walnuts**
- **2 tablespoons of oil**
- **chilli powder**
- **salt**

Chop the garlic and heat it for 1 minute with a little oil and water in a pan. Wash the broccoli, divide them into small pieces and combine them at the base with a bit of salt, oil, ½ glass of water. Leave to simmer for about 15 minutes. Separately, prepare the pasta in plenty of water and when it is cooked, drain and mix it with the broccoli. Serve immediately with a sprinkle of chopped walnuts or, if you prefer, topped with a little Parmesan cheese and a pinch of chili powder.

15) Cabbage rolls with lentils

Ingredients:
- **8 cabbage leaves**
- **300 g of cooked lentils**
- **1 sprig of rosemary**
- **1 bay leaf**
- **bread crumbs**
- **2 cloves of garlic**
- **50 g of shelled walnuts**
- **4 tablespoons of oil**
- **2 tablespoons of soy sauce**
- **salt**

Wash the cabbage and blanch it for a few minutes in a little water. Remove the leaves with a slotted spoon and place them on a cloth. Let them cool down. Mix the lentils with the minced garlic and herbs, then with the ground walnuts and, if needed, little breadcrumbs to compact the filling. Season with salt and add half of the oil. Stir well until you have a homogeneous mixture. Remove the hardest rib of the cabbage. Distribute the filling in the leaves' center, close into a bundle, and tied with a kitchen string. Arrange the rolls in a saucepan; add the bay leaf, rosemary, and soy sauce. Sprinkle with the cabbage cooking water and cook the rolls for about 40 minutes, turning them every so often and pouring more hot liquid if necessary. Finally, season with salt and season with the remaining oil.

Chapter 7: Fish

1)   Crispy salmon

Ingredients:
- **Salmon fillet (4 of 250 g each) 1 kg**
- **Bread 100 g**
- **1 sprig parsley**
- **Dill 1 sprig**
- **Thyme 4 sprigs**
- **Rosemary 2 sprigs**
- **Lemon zest 1**
- **Extra virgin olive oil 50 g**
- **White pepper in grains 1 tsp**
- **Salt up to taste**

First, prepare the breading: cut the bread into pieces and put it in a mixer, then add the dill, the peeled thyme, the needles of rosemary and parsley. Pour in the oil too, then add the lemon zest, salt and white pepper. Blend until you get a coarse consistency. Now take care of the salmon fillets: remove the skin with a thin-bladed knife and remove the bones with the help of a kitchen tongs, then transfer the fillets to a drip pan lined with parchment paper and cover them with the breading, making it adhere well with your hands. . After covering the fillets evenly, cook in a preheated convection oven at 190 ° for about 20 minutes. After the cooking time, take out and serve your crispy salmon hot!

2)   Baked salmon

Ingredients:
- **Salmon steaks (4 pieces) 660 g**
- **Potatoes 170 g**
- **Lemon zest 1**
- **Lemon juice 25 g**
- **Dry white wine 25 g**
- **Extra virgin olive oil 50 g**
- **Parsley to chop 1 tbsp**
- **Salt up to taste**
- **Black pepper to taste**

To prepare the baked salmon, first remove the fish bones with tweezers and check that there are no bones left by sliding a fingertip on the pulp. Remove the spine with a knife, then roll one end on itself and wrap the other end around the slice to obtain a medallion. Tie the medallion with a kitchen string to ensure that it maintains the shape even during cooking and transfer the medallions on a baking sheet lined with parchment paper. Take a fairly regular shaped potato, wash it and cut it into thin slices with a mandolin, without peeling it: the slices must be no more than 1 mm thick otherwise they will not be cooked enough. Now take care of the emulsion: grate the zest of a lemon in a bowl, then add 25 g of lemon juice, oil, white wine, chopped parsley, salt and pepper and mix well with a fork. Season the salmon medallions with part of the emulsion, then cover them with the slightly overlapping potato discs and sprinkle the potatoes with the remaining emulsion. When the medallions are ready, bake in a preheated static oven at 180 ° for about 20 minutes, then operate the grill at 240 ° and continue cooking for another 3-4 minutes, until the potatoes are golden. After the cooking time has elapsed, remove the cooking string and immediately serve your delicious baked salmon!

3) Salmon rice

Ingredients:
- Rice 350 g
- Salmon steaks 250 g
- Leeks 1
- Extra virgin olive oil q.s.
- 1 clove garlic
- ½ glass white wine
- Parmesan to be grated 20 g
- Salt up to taste
- Black pepper to taste
- Fish broth 500 ml

FOR THE FLAVORED BUTTER
- Butter 80 g
- Marjoram 1 sprig
- Dill 1 sprig
- Thyme 1 sprig
- Lemon zest ½
- Salt up to taste

Prepare the flavored butter by chopping the herbs and grating the lemon zest, allow the butter to soften at room temperature and when it has reached a creamy consistency add the chopped herbs, lemon zest and salt. Meanwhile, clean the salmon steak and cut it into small pieces. Heat a tablespoon of oil in a pan with a clove of whole garlic and brown the salmon bites for 2/3 minutes, add salt and set the salmon aside, removing the garlic. Now start preparing the risotto: finely chop the leek and sauté it over low heat with two tablespoons of oil in a pan. Pour in the rice and toast it for a few moments over high heat, stirring with a wooden spoon. Deglaze with the counter wine and continue cooking, stirring occasionally, taking care that the rice does not stick, adding the broth (vegetable or fish) a little at a time. Halfway through cooking add the salmon morsels, season with salt if necessary and when the rice is well cooked, remove it from the heat and stir in the herb-flavored butter and a couple of tablespoons of grated cheese, if you like.

4)   Mediterranean-style salmon fillets

Ingredients:
- **Salmon 800 g**
- **Cherry tomatoes 350 g**
- **Dried oregano 1 sprig**
- **Extra virgin olive oil 30 g**
- **Salt up to taste**
- **1 clove garlic**
- **Pitted black olives 70 g**
- **Pickled capers 5 g**

Start washing the tomatoes, then dry them and cut them into 4. Transfer them to a large bowl, add the peeled and halved garlic and the chopped dried oregano. Add the oil, salt, mix everything and cover with cling film. Let the tomatoes macerate for about 1 hour at room temperature. After this time, take the salmon steak and remove any bones with tweezers and remove the skin if it is present; then cut into 4 fillets of equal thickness. Take back the cherry tomatoes, remove the garlic and transfer them to a lightly greased baking dish. Arrange the salmon fillets on top of the cherry tomatoes and with a teaspoon take some cherry tomatoes and arrange them on top of the salmon. Salt, pepper, add the black olives and capers. Bake in a preheated static oven at 180 ° for about 15 minutes (if you want to use the convection oven, bake at 160 ° for about 10 minutes). After this time, take out and serve your Mediterranean salmon fillets still hot!

5) Tuna tartare

Ingredients:
•Tuna in slices 450 g
•Oranges 1
•Extra virgin olive oil 40 g
•Salt up to taste
•Black pepper to taste
•Shortcrust pastry 230 g
•Wild fennel 3 sprigs

Start grating the zest of an orange, then cut it in half and squeeze the juice. In a bowl, pour the extra virgin olive oil, the orange juice and its zest. Finely chop the fennel, keeping a few strands aside for the final decoration, add it to the mixture and emulsify with a whisk. Meanwhile, prepare the shortcrust pastry shells. Adjust the emulsion with a pinch of pepper and salt. Prepare the shortcrust pastry shells that will be used to make tartare single portions: roll out the shortcrust pastry (you can use a roll of already made shortcrust pastry), cut out 10 circles of about 10 cm in diameter and line 10 round molds with a diameter of 8 cm , after having buttered them. Prick the bottom with the tines of a fork and cook in white, covered with dried legumes as weight, in the oven at 180 degrees for 10-15 minutes. When they are golden, take them out of the oven, let them cool and turn them out. Take the tuna steaks: make sure you have bought especially fish. It is recommended to freeze it for 96 hours at -18 degrees and then defrost it for use in the recipe. Rinse and dry the tuna fillets with absorbent paper. Cut them into small cubes half a centimeter thick and place them in a large bowl. Pour the oil and orange emulsion over them and mix so that the tuna is well flavored. Then fill the cakes with one or two tablespoons of tuna tartare and decorate your tartare with a few sprigs of fennel.

6)   Tuna in pistachio crust

Ingredients:
- **Tuna 600 g**
- **Poppy seeds 1 tbsp**
- **Extra virgin olive oil 3 tbsp**
- **Breadcrumbs 20 g**
- **Chopped pistachios 50**
- **Dried tomatoes in oil 30 g**
- **Salt up to taste**

Get yourself a slice of fresh tuna, place the slice in the freezer for at least an hour so that it is more convenient to cut without breaking the fibers. Remove the tuna from the freezer and cut it lengthwise into slices about 2-3 cm thick. Put the tuna slices in a baking dish and drizzle them with the olive oil. Meanwhile, dry the dried tomatoes with a cloth to remove excess oil and chop finely with a knife. Place the chopped pistachios in a bowl, add the chopped tomatoes, poppy seeds and breadcrumbs. Stir to mix the ingredients well and salt the breading to taste. Take the slices of tuna and pass them in the breadcrumbs, pressing well on all sides. Place a couple of tablespoons of extra virgin olive oil in a non-stick pan and once the necessary heat is reached, add the breaded tuna slices and cook them for 1 minute per side, turning them only once. Do not continue cooking so that the tuna remains pink inside, the tuna must not turn white otherwise the meat will be harder. Remove the pistachio crusted tuna from the pan and cut into 2 cm thick slices, then place them on a serving dish and serve immediately.

7)   Spaghetti with tuna

Ingredients:
•Spaghetti 320 g
•Tuna in oil (drained) 150 g
•Peeled tomatoes 400 g
•Extra virgin olive oil q.s.
•Salt up to taste
•Black pepper to taste
•Basil to taste
•Onions ½

Start by putting a pot full of water on the stove, add salt to taste when boiling: it will be used for cooking the pasta. Drain the tuna fillet from the conservation oil. Meanwhile, peel the onion, slice it thinly. Heat the olive oil in a pan and add the sliced onion. Let it dry over low heat for a few minutes, stirring often; fray the tuna with your hands and add it to the pan when the onion is soft and let it brown for a couple of minutes, stirring constantly. Now, mash the tomatoes with a fork and pour them into the pan with the tuna; let the sauce cook for about 10 minutes. Meanwhile, cook the spaghetti, while the pasta is cooking, the sauce will also be ready. Drain the spaghetti directly into the pan with the tuna, season with the ground pepper, turn off the heat and perfume with the fresh basil leaves. Stir and serve your tuna spaghetti hot!

8)   Tuna glazed with soy sauce

Ingredients:
- **Tuna fillet 400 g**
- **Red cabbage 500 g**
- **Soy sauce 50 g**
- **White wine vinegar 100 g**
- **Salt up to 30 g**
- **Extra virgin olive oil 20 g**
- **Basil 4 leaves**
- **Sesame seeds 30 g**

Start with the vegetables: julienne the cabbage and place it in a bowl, sprinkling with white wine vinegar and seasoning with salt. Mix the ingredients well and leave to macerate for at least 1 hour, covering with cling film. After this time, drain and rinse the cabbage thoroughly under plenty of running water. Then cook it in a non-stick pan in which you have heated 15 g of oil. Flavored with well washed and dried basil leaves and cover with a lid, cooking over low heat for about 10 minutes. When cooked, the cabbage should still be crunchy. While the cabbage is cooking, dedicate yourself to the tuna. Take a small bowl and pour the soy sauce. Take care of the tuna: make sure you have a fillet already cut down; we advise you to freeze the fillet for at least 96 hours at -18 degrees and then defrost for preparation. Cut the tuna into slices about 4 cm thick. Then place a small bowl next to the soy sauce in which you will have poured the white sesame seeds. Take a slice of tuna and wet it on all sides with the soy sauce, then completely cover the long sides of the tuna slice with sesame seeds. Repeat the operation with all the slices of tuna. Now take a non-stick pan and pour in 5 g of oil: heat it up and place the slices of tuna on the long sides. Blanch the tuna slices for about 2 minutes, then flip them to cook them on the other side for another 2 minutes. For even cooking, you can also sear the tuna slices sideways, 1 minute on each side. Place a bed of cabbage on the serving dish and arrange the slices of tuna on top of it, accompanying with the soy sauce. Your tuna glazed with soy sauce is then ready to be brought to the table and enjoyed!

9) Baked sardines

Ingredients:
- **18 sardines for a total of about 250 g**
- **Breadcrumbs 60 g**
- **Extra virgin olive oil 60 g**
- **1 sprig parsley**
- **Thyme 1 sprig**
- **1 clove garlic**
- **Grated Parmesan cheese 20 g**
- **Pine nuts 30 g**
- **Extra virgin olive oil to grease the pan 15g**

Pour the breadcrumbs, grated cheese and the crushed garlic clove into a bowl. Rinse, dry and finely chop the parsley; then also add it to the breading and further flavor with the thyme leaves; pour the 60 g of oil and mix everything until you get a uniform mixture. At this point take a baking dish measuring 19x15 cm and sprinkle it with about 15 g of oil. Arrange the sardines horizontally without overlapping each other, salt (not excessively), pepper and cover with half of the previously prepared mixture. Arrange another layer of sardines, taking care to position them vertically (opposite to before), salt, pepper and cover the entire surface with the remaining part of the breading. Finish by decorating the surface with pine nuts. Then cook the sardines in the oven in grill mode at 200 ° for 8 minutes, until they are golden brown. Once cooked, serve the baked sardines while still hot.

10) Spaghetti with anchovies and breadcrumbs

Ingredients:
- **Spaghetti 320 g**
- **Anchovies in oil 30 g**
- **Extra virgin olive oil 20 g**
- **Breadcrumbs 70 g**
- **3 cloves garlic**

Put a pan with water on the heat and bring to a boil: it will then be used to cook the pasta. Meanwhile, pour 10 g of extra virgin olive oil into a pan, then add the peeled garlic cloves and the anchovy fillets drained from the preservation oil. Peel a ladle of hot water and pour it into the pan, so you can melt the anchovies in the best possible way. This will take about 10 minutes so stir often. Meanwhile, in a separate pan pour 10 g of extra virgin olive oil, then add breadcrumbs to toast it and mix everything until the crumbs are golden; keep aside. At this point, cook the pasta in boiling water; you can add at most very little coarse salt if you prefer, as anchovies are very tasty. Cook the spaghetti for the time indicated on the package. After the time has elapsed, remove the garlic cloves from the saucepan and drain the pasta by dipping it directly into the pan. Add some of the breadcrumbs and mix. If necessary, add a little more cooking water, then serve your spaghetti with the anchovies and garnish with a final sprinkling of breadcrumbs.

11) Orange mackerel

Ingredients:
- Mackerel (4 whole clean) 1200 g
- Orange peel 1
- Extra virgin olive oil q.s.

FOR MARINATING
- Orange juice
- Extra virgin olive oil 30 g
- Dill 2 sprigs
- 2 cloves garlic
- Black peppercorns 1 tbsp
- Salt up to 1 tbsp

Make diagonal cuts on the sides of the mackerel and set aside. Take care of the ingredients for the marinade: with the back of the spoon, crush the peppercorns so they will release their aroma better, then squeeze the juice from the oranges. Peel and thinly slice the garlic. Grease a baking dish with oil, place the mackerel on top and season them on the surface with another drizzle of oil, the peppercorns, salt, scented with the sprigs of dill and flavored with the slices of garlic. Finally, sprinkle the fish with half of the orange juice, cover with plastic wrap and leave to marinate for 2 hours in the refrigerator. After the marinating time, go to cooking: heat a pan with a drizzle of olive oil and, when it is hot, lay the fillets. Let them cook over high heat for 4 minutes without touching them, then turn them, sprinkle them with the remaining orange juice and continue cooking for another 2 minutes. Once the sauce has congealed and the mackerel are well flavored, serve them immediately garnishing them with grated orange zest on the surface.

12) Mackerel in foil

Ingredients:
- **Mackerel (2 clean mackerel)**
- **Celery 90 g**
- **Yellow peppers 70 g**
- **Tomatoes 60 g**
- **Eggplant 50 g**
- **Lemons 1**
- **Basil to taste**
- **Extra virgin olive oil q.s.**
- **Black pepper to taste**
- **Salt up to taste**

Chop the celery and cut it into cubes, then cut the eggplants into slices and cut into cubes. Remove the internal seeds and the stalk of the pepper and cut it first into strips and then into cubes. Finally, cut the tomatoes into cubes. Transfer all the cut vegetables to a bowl, scented with fresh basil leaves and season with oil, salt and pepper. Now place each clean mackerel on a 35x31 cm sheet of parchment paper, fill the belly of the mackerel with a spoonful of vegetables and then distribute the rest around the fish. Season the fish with a drizzle of olive oil. Wash the lemon and cut into thin slices, then place 3 lemon slices on top of each mackerel. Now close the parcel by lifting the flaps of parchment paper and placing them on top of the fish, then seal well by folding the sides. Place the packets on a baking tray lined with parchment paper and bake in a preheated static oven at 200 ° for 20 minutes. When cooked, take your mackerel in foil out of the oven and serve hot.

13) Swordfish with tomato sauce

Ingredients:
- Swordfish (2 slices) 400 g
- Lemons 1
- Marjoram 3 sprigs
- Extra virgin olive oil 30 g
- Salt up to taste
- Black pepper to taste

FOR THE TOMATO SAUCE
- Tomatoes 250 g
- Worcestershire sauce 20 ml
- 1 clove garlic
- Extra virgin olive oil 15 g
- Salt up to taste
- Black pepper to taste

First, take care of the marinade: place the swordfish fillet in a fairly large baking dish, add the oil, the marjoram leaves, the grated rind of a lemon (keep some aside for the final garnish) and the juice. of half a lemon. Turn the fish on both sides to make sure it is evenly flavored, then cover the dish with cling film and set it aside temporarily. Wash the cherry tomatoes and cut them in half; Heat the oil in a pan, add the garlic clove and let it brown briefly. Add the cherry tomatoes, salt, pepper and mix. Then deglaze with the Worcestershire sauce. Let the cherry tomatoes cook for 10 minutes over medium heat, stirring occasionally. Once cooked, turn off the heat, remove the garlic and transfer them to a tall, narrow container, then blend them with an immersion blender until you get a smooth and homogeneous sauce. Heat another pan well, remove the swordfish from the marinade and place it in the pan, add salt and sear the fish over medium-high heat for 2 minutes on one side and for 1 minute on the other. Once cooked, transfer the swordfish to a plate and cut into cubes. At this point you can assemble the serving dishes: sprinkle the bottom with a little tomato sauce, add the swordfish morsels and finally garnish with a few leaves of marjoram, the lemon zest that you had kept aside and a minced pepper: your swordfish with tomato sauce is ready to be served!

14) Swordfish carpaccio with green and pink pepper

Ingredients:
- **Swordfish 500**
- **Semi-skimmed milk 250 g**
- **Pink peppercorns 5**
- **Green peppercorns 10**
- **Extra virgin olive oil 50 g**
- **Himalayan salt (pink) 5 g**

Start by cutting the swordfish slices. Cut the swordfish steak into 16 slices of about 30 g each and 3-4 mm thick. To facilitate the operation, keep the swordfish steak to compact it in the freezer for an hour before slicing it. If you don't have a slicer available, buy the swordfish already cut into slices for the carpaccio or have it cut in your trusted fish shop. Remove the skin of the swordfish with a knife and arrange the slices in a baking dish. Start preparing the marinade: pour the milk and oil into a bowl. Add the green peppercorns, pink pepper and pink Himalayan salt. Emulsify the mixture with a whisk to mix all the ingredients. Pour the marinade into the pan where you have placed the swordfish slices and cover with plastic wrap. The carpaccio must marinate in the refrigerator for at least 4 hours. After this time, remove the swordfish carpaccio from the fridge and, with the help of a spatula, lift the slices of swordfish one by one, draining the marinade a little, and place them in an ovenproof dish. Bake at 180 degrees for no more than 5 minutes, so that the the fish releases the absorbed marinade. Stir in the swordfish carpaccio with green and pink pepper before serving.

15) Cod fillet with ginger

Ingredients:
- Cod fillet 400 g
- Salt up to taste
- Black pepper to taste
- Extra virgin olive oil 50 g
- Lime zest 1
- Lime juice 10 g
- Fresh ginger (pulp) 20 g
- Mint a few leaves

FOR THE RICE
- Basmati rice 200 g
- Coconut milk 400 g
- Water 200 g
- Coarse salt 1 tbsp
- Cinnamon sticks 1
- Curry 1 tsp

Grate the lime zest in a bowl and squeeze it into juice and pour 10 g into the same bowl. Peel the ginger and grate it, then collect the pulp with a spoon and place it in the bowl with the lime, pour in the olive oil and stir to mix the sauce. Take the cod fillets and place them on a baking sheet lined with parchment paper, salt them and spread the sauce on the surface. Bake in a preheated static oven at 220 ° for 25 minutes. Meanwhile, prepare the rice: pour the basmati rice into a pan, add the coconut milk, the coarse salt, the curry and a stick of cinnamon. Pour in the water, cover with the lid and bring to a boil, then lower the heat and cook for 15 minutes until the liquids are completely absorbed. When the rice has absorbed the liquids, turn off the heat and remove the cinnamon stick. Meanwhile, the cod will be cooked, take it out of the oven and serve it accompanied with the spiced basmati rice, garnishing with mint leaves.

Chapter 8: Salads&Soups

1) Barley and bean soup

Ingredients:
- **200 g of cooked beans**
- **150 g of pearl barley**
- **1 small onion**
- **1 small carrot**
- **1 stalk of celery**
- **100 g approx. of pumpkin pulp**
- **1 sprig of parsley**
- **1 clove of garlic**
- **4 tablespoons of oil**
- **1 pinch of chilli**
- **salt**

Boil the barley in 400 ml of water with a pinch of salt, for about 40 minutes, in a covered pot. Prepare a mixture of garlic, onion, celery, carrot, and parsley; cut the pumpkin into cubes. Fry the mixture in oil in a large pot with a pinch of salt; then add the pumpkin and let it simmer for five minutes, until softened, possibly with a little water. Then add the barley and beans with their cooking water or a little broth to get the right consistency (the soup should be creamy); bring to a boil and cook for another 5 minutes. Season with a pinch of chili and serve hot. Alternatively, you can cook the barley directly with the vegetables and add the beans towards cooking.

2)   Cream of spinach with pine nuts

Ingredients:
- 1 kg of spinach
- 2 shallots
- 500 ml of vegetable broth
- 100 ml of soy milk
- 100 g of tofu
- 2 tablespoons of flour
- 2 tablespoons of pine nuts
- 2 teaspoons of turmeric
- 2 tablespoons of oil
- salt and pepper

Clean the spinach, wash and drain them. Finely chop the shallots and let them soften in a saucepan with a little broth for about ten minutes. Add the flour, stir so that it does not form lumps, and add the spinach. Add salt, stir briefly and pour in the warmed milk and remaining broth, tofu, and turmeric. Cook for about ten minutes and blend by immersion. Peppered, seasoned with oil, and served garnished with lightly toasted pine nuts and, if desired, with oatcakes.

3) Chestnut and chickpea soup

Ingredients:
- **200 g of dried chestnuts**
- **200 g of chickpeas**
- **2 tablespoons of chopped parsley**
- **1 teaspoon of dried thyme**
- **1 clove of garlic**
- **2 shallots**
- **4 tablespoons of dry white wine**
- **1 teaspoon of fennel seeds**
- **1 bay leaf**
- **1 chilli**
- **3 tablespoons of oil**
- **salt**

Soak chickpeas and chestnuts separately for one night. Drain and rinse them. Put the first courses in a pressure cooker with the bay leaf and garlic. Cover them with water and cook for 15 minutes from the whistle. As soon as possible, carefully open the pot, add the chestnuts and then the fennel seeds and salt. Continue the pressure cooking for another 15 minutes. Meanwhile, peel and chop the shallots with the chilli. Sauté them in a pan with the thyme and wine. As soon as they begin to smell, turn them off and add them to the contents of the pot, which you will always have uncovered with caution. Continue cooking for another 10 minutes. Remove the bay leaf and blend almost all the chickpeas and chestnuts, using hot water if needed. Season with salt and season with oil. Serve the soup hot.

4)   Spiced pumpkin cream

Ingredients:
- **1.5 kg of pumpkin**
- **1 shallot**
- **vegetable broth or water to taste**
- **1 teaspoon of curry powder**
- **3 cloves**
- **2 slices of fresh ginger**
- **Salt to taste.**
- **extra virgin olive oil as needed**

Finely chop the shallot and set it aside. Prepare the fresh ginger by cutting two rounds from the root, remove the peel, and cut them coarsely. Also, prepare the other spices required by the recipe for use. In the meantime, wash the pumpkin and cut it into medium sized pieces without removing the skin. Put the already prepared vegetable broth on the fire (even just the water is fine) and put it to heat so that it is already hot when we add it to the pumpkin. Put a saucepan with two tablespoons of extra virgin olive oil and half a coffee glass of water on the stove: add the shallot, ginger, cloves, and curry. Sauté gently for a few minutes, stirring often. At this point, add the pumpkin cut into pieces, brown it in a pot for a few seconds, add the salt and mix well. Add the vegetable broth or water until it is covered. Cook over high heat for about 20 minutes, add salt, and turn off. Remove the cloves and proceed with an immersion blender, blending the mixture until a soft and velvety cream is obtained. Serve hot with a drizzle of raw oil, a sprinkling of toasted sesame seeds, and croutons.

5)   Pumpkin and walnut rice salad

Ingredients:
- 100 g of cooked brown rice
- 200 g of grated pumpkin
- 1 apple
- 10 walnut kernels
- 1 handful of mustard sprouts
- 2 tablespoons of oil
- 1 tablespoon of wine vinegar
- pepper
- salt

It is a recipe that lends itself to recycling previously cooked rice or other grains. Season the brown rice with crumbled walnut kernels. Apart from washing and peeling an apple and pumpkin. Prepare a diced apple and pumpkin to sauté in a pan in a little oil and a salt pinch. Transfer the seasoning to a bowl with the rice and walnuts and season everything with oil, vinegar, and ground pepper. To close, distribute the mustard sprouts evenly.

6)   Autumn garden soup

Ingredients:
- 1 small leek
- 2 cloves of minced garlic
- 2 tablespoons of minced ginger
- 100 g of celeriac
- 200 g of carrots
- 200 g of potatoes
- 100 g of beetroot
- about 1 l of vegetable broth
- 2 tablespoons of chives
- 1 teaspoon of oil
- salt

Cut the leek in half lengthwise and then into small pieces; the other diced vegetables. Sauté the leek for a few minutes in the oil with a pinch of salt over low heat; add half of the garlic and ginger, cook for a minute. Put the other vegetables in the pot and let it all flavor; then pour in the broth and a nice pinch of salt, bring to a boil and cook covered, simmering over low heat for about 30 minutes. Before serving, sprinkle with the remaining minced garlic and ginger. Garnish the individual portions of soup with finely chopped chives.

7) Cream of corn

Ingredients:
- **450 g of sweet corn**
- **1 small white onion**
- **380 g of potatoes**
- **1 teaspoon of vegetable butter**
- **300 ml of vegetable broth**
- **350 ml of oat milk**
- **1 lime**
- **White pepper**

To garnish
- **slices of avocado**
- **parsley leaves**

In a high-sided saucepan, soften the butter and brown the onion and peeled potatoes cut into small cubes for 5 minutes, stirring and making sure they do not burn. Then add the drained corn, the vegetable broth, and the oat milk. Bring slowly to a boil, lightly salt, and cook for 30 minutes. After this time, purée everything with a fine-texture vegetable mill, helping with the cooking liquid. The filter will only have to retain the well-pressed skins, especially those of the corn kernels. Otherwise, the flavor will be lost. Stir in the lime juice and make the cream homogeneous. Serve it in bowls decorated with a thin slice of avocado and a sprinkle of pepper; give the final touch with a leaf of parsley.

8)   Red rice salad

Ingredients:
- **1 cup of red rice**
- **150 g of cooked beans**
- **½ bunch of spring onions**
- **2 sticks of celery**
- **2 carrots**
- **½ cup of corn**
- **2 tablespoons of pitted green olives**
- **1 tablespoon of salted capers**
- **parsley**
- **basil**
- **oil**
- **lemon juice**
- **salt**

Wash the rice and cook it with a cup and a half of water and a pinch of salt. Dice the carrots, celery, and the white part of the spring onions. Blanch them separately in boiling water with a pinch of salt for a few minutes so that they remain crunchy, then let them drain. Soak the capers to desalt them, changing the water several times. Cut the olives into rings. Chop the green part of the spring onions, capers, and aromatic herbs. When the rice has cooled, mix it with the beans, corn and other ingredients already prepared. Dress with oil and lemon juice. Let it rest for a couple of hours before serving.

9)   Spelled with avocado, orange and capers

Ingredients:
- **250 g of peeled spelled**
- **1 small avocado**
- **1 orange**
- **2 small handfuls of salted capers**
- **oil, to taste**
- **the juice of ½ lemon**
- **whole sea salt, to taste**
- **dried oregano, to taste**
- **white pepper, to taste**

Wash the spelled under cold running water and drain it. Cook it for about 45 minutes in filtered water, over low heat and with a lid, using 2 parts of water for one cereal part. Drain it and let it cool. In the meantime, clean the avocado, cut it into small pieces, peel the orange, divide it into raw peeled wedges, and then cut them into small pieces. Soak the capers in filtered water for 10-15 minutes, then rinse and squeeze them well. Add the already cooked spelled, cold or at room temperature, the avocado, the orange, and the capers in a salad bowl. Season with extra virgin olive oil, lemon juice, and salt, add the dried, chopped oregano and freshly ground pepper, and mix well. Serve immediately, or keep the spelled salad in the refrigerator until ready to serve.

10) Chickpea and rice soup

Ingredients:
- **250 g of chickpeas**
- **100 g of brown rice**
- **1 onion**
- **2 carrots**
- **2 sticks of celery**
- **1 tomato**
- **2 tablespoons of oil**
- **salt and pepper**

Soak the chickpeas for 24 hours, changing the liquid from time to time. In the end, rinse them and put them in a pressure cooker just covered with cold water. Cook them for 10-15 minutes, starting from the whistle. At this point, continue cooking as normal. After 10-15 minutes, add the rice first and the sliced onion and celery, the diced carrots, the chopped tomato, or the concentrate dissolved in hot water. Salt. If necessary, add more hot liquid. When the cereal and legumes are ready, season the soup with oil and pepper.

11) Broccoli cream

Ingredients:
- **400 g of broccoli**
- **1 potato**
- **100 ml of oat milk**
- **2 tablespoons of oil**
- **chilli powder, to taste**
- **sea salt to taste**

Clean the broccoli, divide them into florets and steam them, keeping their cooking water. Wash, peel, and steam the potato as well. Once cooked, pour the broccoli into the bowl of a mixer. Add about 200ml of their cooking water, the cooked potato, the oat milk, the oil, salt, and blend until you get the desired consistency. Increase the doses of water or milk if necessary. Before serving, reheat the cream if it has cooled in the meantime. Divide into individual bowls or serving plates, complete with a drizzle of oil and chili to taste and serve.

12) Creamy red lentil and pumpkin soup

Ingredients:
- **300 g of lentils**
- **1 small onion**
- **300 g of pumpkin**
- **2 bay leaves**
- **1 tablespoon of oil**
- **750 ml of water**
- **1 tablespoon of white miso**
- **parsley**
- **1 pinch of salt**

Cut the onion and pumpkin into cubes. Heat the oil in a saucepan and sauté the onion with a pinch of salt, stirring for a few minutes; then add the pumpkin, bay leaf, lentils, and water. Bring to a boil and cook gently for 30-40 minutes. In the last 5 minutes of cooking, add the miso diluted with a little hot broth. Serve with chopped parsley garnish.

Chapter 9: Dessert

1) Spiced apple pie

Ingredients:
- **3 apples**
- **200 g of spelled flour type 0**
- **30 g of corn starch**
- **50 g of raisins**
- **50 g of peeled and chopped almonds**
- **150-200 ml of almond or soy milk**
- **120 ml of concentrated apple juice**
- **50 ml of corn oil**
- **½ teaspoon of cinnamon**
- **½ teaspoon of vanilla**
- **1 pinch of clove powder**
- **the grated zest of ½ lemon**
- **½ sachet of baking powder**
- **1 pinch of salt**

Cut the apples into small pieces, soak the raisins. In a bowl, mix the flour, starch, almonds, spices, lemon peel, salt, and yeast; in another, milk, concentrated juice, oil, apples, and drained raisins. Mix all the ingredients, transfer the mixture into a pan lined with parchment paper and bake at 190 ° for about 45 minutes. Check the cooking with a toothpick before serving.

2) Carrot cake

Ingredients:
- 200 g of wholemeal flour
- 80 g of almonds
- 80 g of raisins
- 200 g of carrots
- 100 g of rice malt
- 4 tablespoons of sunflower oil
- 1 orange
- 3 tablespoons of corn starch
- 1 teaspoon of yeast
- ½ teaspoon of natural vanilla
- soya milk
- 1 pinch of salt

Wash the orange, grate the zest and squeeze the juice. Put the first in a bowl together with the flour, finely ground almonds, starch, yeast, vanilla, and salt. Stir. Mix the oil, malt, and orange juice in a bowl. Gradually add them to the dry ingredients. Complete with grated carrots and rinsed raisins. If the dough is too firm, dilute it with a little soy milk. Line a square mold of about 20 cm on each side with baking paper. Transfer the mixture, level it, and bake at 180 degrees for about 45 minutes. Check the cooking with a toothpick, which must come out dry. Let the cake cool in the pan, turn it out of the mold, and let it cool.

3) Banana dessert

Ingredients:
- 50 g of pitted dates
- 10 g of sultanas
- 100 g of Pecan nuts
- 50 g of peeled almonds
- 50 g of Rapè coconut
- Himalayan salt
- 1 tablespoon of orange juice
- 1 tablespoon of coconut oil
- cinnamon powder

For the stuffing
- 2 large bananas
- 420 g of cashews soaked for about 6-7 hours
- the juice and grated zest of ½ organic lemon
- 150 ml of agave syrup, cooled in the freezer for about 25 minutes
- 150 g of cocoa butter
- 1 tablespoon of coconut oil

To garnish
- ½ bar of dark chocolate or maple syrup or chopped hazelnuts
- banana slices (optional)

Wash the dates and raisins under running water, then chop them finely in a mixer; without turning off the appliance, add the salt, orange juice, coconut oil, and cinnamon. When you have obtained a compact mixture, add the Pecan nuts and the chopped almonds in thin grains separately, complete with the Rapè coconut. Mix the dough well and roll it out on the bottom of a small cake pan (or a loaf pan), which you will have lined with baking paper. Level it well on the surface using a spatula and put it to solidify in the freezer or refrigerator.

Drain the cashews and grind them for a long time in the mixer to make them doughy. Continuing to operate, first add the lemon juice and zest, agave syrup, cocoa butter, and melted coconut oil; then add the bananas and continue until you have a soft cream. Pour it on the cooled base and place it in the freezer, so that it becomes firm. You can also divide it into individual portions. Let it cool for a few minutes before serving. Decorate with a few banana slices, if you like, or with dark chocolate cut into flakes or with maple syrup and chopped hazelnuts.

4) Almond and apricot cake

Ingredients:
- **500g of chopped apricots + other ripe ones for garnish**
- **½ cup of chopped dried apricots**
- **2 tablespoons of agar-agar**
- **2 cups of almond milk**
- **2 tablespoons of almond cream**
- **the grated zest of ½ lemon**
- **1 teaspoon of vanilla**
- **4 tablespoons of corn starch**
- **½ cup of concentrated apple juice**
- **200 g of ladyfingers**
- **Apple juice**
- **salt**

Put the fresh and dried apricots in a pot together with half a cup of water, the agar-agar, and a pinch of salt. Stirring constantly, bring to a boil, and cook for 5-10 minutes. When cooked, add the concentrated juice, then blend. Use a little almond milk to dissolve the corn starch and rest on the heat with a pinch of salt, lemon peel, and vanilla. When it is about to boil, remove it from the stove, add the almond cream and starch, and then let it boil again and turn it off. Blend the apricots, add the cream and adjust the flavor by adding, if necessary, more concentrated apple juice. Cut the ladyfingers at one end and quickly dip them in the apple juice. Arrange them standing along the edge of a mold of about 22 cm and distribute the cutouts on the bottom. Cover with the apricot cream and leave to cool for a few hours. Remove the hinge from the mold and serve the cake decorated with some halved fresh apricots.

5) Strawberry tartlets

Ingredients:
For the shortcrust pastry
- **250 g of wholemeal flour**
- **50 g of coconut butter**
- **2 tablespoons of rice flour**
- **2 tablespoons of brown sugar**
- **1 teaspoon of ground cinnamon**
- **1 pinch of pink salt**

For coverage
- **4 tablespoons of unsweetened apricot jam**
- **2 tablespoons of chopped hazelnuts**
- **½ tablespoon of lemon juice**
- **1 tablespoon of cherry, plum or apricot distillate**
- **400 g of strawberries**
- **1 sprig of mint**

Melt the coconut butter in a double boiler and let it cool. Pour it into the mixer with the other ingredients and sugar. Operate; when large crumbs begin to form, add a few tablespoons of cold water at a time, continuing to knead the dough until it collects into a ball. Wrap it in a cloth and put it in the fridge for 30 minutes.

It is using a damp brush, grease 8 molds with a diameter of 10 cm with oil. Obtain from the thinly rolled dough as many discs large enough to cover the molds' walls and the bottom. They will have to adhere everywhere. Prick the bottom with a fork. Cover each tart with a piece of parchment paper and a few dried beans. Bake at 180 degrees for 15 minutes, remove the paper and the legumes, cook them for another 5 minutes. After another ten minutes, remove them, and once cold, unmold them. Heat the jam with the distillate until it is shiny. Turn off and add the lemon juice. After a few minutes, brush part of the mixture on the bases. Wash the strawberries, dry them gently and slice them not too thin. Distribute them over the dough. Cover with the remaining jam, sprinkle the surface with the grains, and let it rest in a cool place for about an hour. Just before serving, garnish the tarts with mint leaves.

6)   Chocolate with avocado and orange

Ingredients:
- **200 g of pitted dates soaked for 15 minutes**
- **150 g of walnut kernels**
- **150 g of white almonds**
- **1 tablespoon of orange juice**
- **1 tablespoon of coconut oil**
- **½ teaspoon of sea salt**

For the stuffing
- **5 large ripe avocados, peeled**
- **100 g of coconut oil**
- **1 tablespoon of white almond cream**
- **50 g of melted cocoa butter**
- **the grated zest of ½ orange**
- **½ teaspoon of vanilla powder**
- **170 g of cocoa powder**
- **250 g of agave syrup**

To garnish
- **dark chocolate grains**

Soak the dates for 15 minutes. Let the maple syrup cool in the freezer for about 25 minutes. Finely grind the walnuts and almonds in the bowl of a mixer. Keep them aside. In their place, put the drained dates and purée them. Then, continuing to operate the appliance, add the salt, coconut oil, orange juice, and the previously prepared grains. When you have a compact mixture, the spread is based on a pan (or a loaf pan) lined with baking paper. Level it well with a spatula and remove it in the freezer or in the refrigerator to make it firm. Gather all the ingredients required for the filling in a mixer and start. You will need to get a well blended mixture. Pour on the solidified base and pass the cake in the refrigerator or freezer so that it hardens. Decorated with one of the proposed alternatives and served.

7) Chocolate nut and almond balls

Ingredients:
- **200 g of wholemeal flour**
- **150 g of walnuts**
- **50 g of pine nuts**
- **50 g of sunflower seeds**
- **200 g of almonds**
- **50 g of flax seeds**
- **100 g of raisins**
- **100 g of dark chocolate in small pieces**
- **400 g of rice malt**
- **1 lemon**
- **1 orange**
- **6 tablespoons of brown sugar**

Soak the raisins in warm water. In the meantime, grate the peel of a lemon and an organic orange and place them in a large bowl. Add the coarsely chopped walnuts and almonds, flax seeds, sunflower seeds, and pine nuts. Stir in the flour, chocolate, and squeezed raisins and mix well with your hands. Then add the malt and continue to mix all the ingredients with energy. Lightly moisten your hands and form medium-sized balls that you will arrange quite far from each other in a baking tray lined with baking paper. Bake for about 10-12 minutes at 180 °. Let cool before serving. Excellent served accompanied by a fragrant compote of apples and spices.

8) Chocolate truffles

Ingredients:
- **100 g of dark chocolate**
- **100 g of almonds**
- **50 g of hazelnuts**
- **100 g of dates**
- **50 g of bitter cocoa**

Soak the almonds in a glass jar for at least 3 hours, then add the dates and leave them for another hour. Meanwhile, heat the dark chocolate in a bain-marie. Drain and set aside the almond and date water. We combine the melted chocolate in the jar with the dried fruit and work it all with the hand blender. Incorporate the chopped hazelnuts and place them in the fridge for an hour. If the mixture is too hard, wet it with one or two tablespoons of soaking liquid. We sprinkle the cocoa on a saucer. We take small doses of the mixture and let them fall on the cocoa. We form balls and compact them well, trying to press them as much as possible. Let's put them in small bowls and skewer each ball with a wooden stick.

9)   Cocoa pudding

Ingredients:
- **500 ml of soy milk**
- **4 tablespoons of unsweetened cocoa**
- **3-4 tablespoons of brown sugar**
- **2 tablespoons of corn starch**
- **1 pinch of natural vanilla**
- **1 pinch of ground cinnamon**
- **chopped hazelnuts to decorate**

Sift the cocoa, starch, and sugar; collect them in a saucepan together with cinnamon and vanilla. First, add 100 ml of milk, stirring well to remove all lumps, and then the rest. Over medium heat, bring to a boil without stopping stirring. Lower the heat and cook for a couple of minutes more until the mixture has thickened. Moisten four single-portion molds and pour the pudding. Let it cool down and put it in the fridge until completely cooled. Decorate with the grains and serve.

10) Baked stuffed apples

Ingredients:
- **6 apples**
- **1 orange**
- **¾ cup of shelled walnuts**
- **¾ cup of raisins**
- **¼ cup of natural apple juice**
- **1 tablespoon of miso**

Wash and with a knife, starting from the top of the apple, make room for the filling. Heat the oven to 150 °. Rinse the raisins and chop them with the walnuts. Wash the orange and finely grate the zest. Add the orange zest, miso, and a teaspoon to the raisin and nut mixture. Mix well. Stuff the apples with the dough. Arrange the apples in a baking dish. Pierce them with a fork all around so that they do not explode during cooking. Pour the apple and orange juice into the pan and bake in the oven for half an hour. Eat them warm or cold.

11) Soft cakes of hazelnuts and apples

Ingredients:
- **200 g of peeled and toasted hazelnuts**
- **100 g of corn flour**
- **80 g of cane sugar**
- **1 apple**
- **2 tablespoons of oil**
- **2 eggs**
- **1 tablespoon of cinnamon powder**
- **1 pinch of salt**

Finely pulverize the hazelnuts in a food processor together with the brown sugar. Transfer the mixture to a bowl and add the peeled apple cut into small pieces, eggs, cinnamon, oil, and salt. Work the ingredients well until a homogeneous mixture is formed. Enclosing it between two spoons, form about 14-15 quenelles that you will place on a baking sheet lined with baking paper. Bake in a preheated oven at 180 degrees for 20-25 minutes. Put the sweets on a plate and let them cool.

12) Bavarian yogurt with pumpkin

Ingredients:
- **350 ml of natural yogurt**
- **150 g of grated pumpkin**
- **50 g of almonds**
- **1 tablespoon of honey**
- **1 tablespoon of agar-agar**
- **1 pinch of salt**

Put the almonds in a pan and toast them for a minute in the oven, shaking the container often. Let them cool before chopping them. Pour the pumpkin into a saucepan with 100 ml of yogurt, salt, and agar-agar; cook for 5 minutes. Remove from heat, let cool and add the remaining yogurt, chopped almonds, honey (or sugar). Stir the mixture well, then pour it into the bowls and let it cool to room temperature or in the refrigerator.

13) Orange cake

Ingredients:
- **300 g of wheat flour 00**
- **150 g of clear raw cane sugar**
- **½ sachet of yeast**
- **the zest and juice of an orange**
- **50 ml of extra virgin olive oil**
- **vanilla sugar to taste**

In a bowl, mix flour, brown sugar, yeast, the grated rind of an orange together with its juice, extra virgin olive oil, and about 100 ml of water. Mix everything with an electric or hand whisk until you get a creamy mixture. Transfer to a pan greased with oil and sprinkled with flour. Bake at 180 degrees for half an hour. When cooked, spread the icing sugar over the cake.

14) Pear cream tart

Ingredients:
300 g of flour
120 ml of soy milk
4 tablespoons of sunflower oil
4 tablespoons of rice malt
the grated zest of 1/2 lemon
1 pinch of salt
1 teaspoon of yeast

For the compote
4 pears
2 dried apricots
1 pinch of salt
1 piece of cinnamon stick
1 clove
2 tablespoons of apple juice

For the cream
500 ml of almond milk
4 tablespoons of agave sap
2 pieces of lemon zest
2 tablespoons of cornstarch
1 teaspoon of starch

Mix the flour, zest, salt, and yeast; gradually sprinkle them with the oil, malt, and milk beaten well with a whisk in another container. Quickly work the mixture on the table and let it rest in the fridge for 30 minutes. Roll it out into a thin disc that you will place in a tart mold. Prick the base with a fork, cover it with baking paper and a few beans. Bake for 15 minutes at 180 degrees. After removing the paper and beans, set them aside. Peel and cut the pears into cubes; mix them in a small saucepan with the apricots cut into small pieces, the clove, the salt, and the cinnamon. Pour in the apple juice and cook the fruit until it is slightly soft. Remove the stick (which you will use for the cream) and the clove. When the compote is warm, distribute it on the pastry. Bake again for 10 minutes, then let cool. Bring 400 ml of milk to the boil with the zest and cinnamon. Dilute the starch and the starch in the remainder. Remove the aromas and add the thickeners, always stirring. Simmer for two minutes and turn off. Sweeten with agave sap. Serve the cream lukewarm with the tart.

15) Cannoli with ricotta and hazelnut

Ingredients:
- **150 g of kamut flour**
- **120 g of ricotta**
- **150 g of hazelnuts**
- **1 egg**
- **the juice and zest of ½ lemon**
- **rice milk**
- **4 tablespoons of coconut sugar**
- **½ teaspoon of vanilla**
- **1 teaspoon of yeast**
- **1 pinch of pink salt**

Gather the flour, 1 tablespoon of sugar, vanilla, salt, and yeast in a bowl. Separately, mash the ricotta with a fork and add half of it to the mixture. Start working the ingredients, helping yourself in the case with a little rice milk. You will need to obtain a firm and homogeneous mixture. Leave it aside while you take care of the filling. Finely chop the hazelnuts, mix them with the rest of the sugar and ricotta, the lemon zest, and the beaten egg. Stir well. Dilute if necessary with a little milk. Roll out the dough with a rolling pin to a thickness of 3 mm. Make six rectangles of the same size. Distribute a small filling in the center of each one and roll the cannolo on itself. Arrange the sweets on a baking sheet lined with baking paper. Brush them on the surface with a little milk and bake them at 180 ° for 30 minutes. Let them cool, take them out of the oven, and place them on a wire rack to cool.

Chapter 10: Sauces, toppings and condiments

1) Spiced pumpkin jam

Ingredients:
- **1 kg of pumpkin**
- **3 tablespoons of 100% malt rice**
- **1 cup of almonds**
- **2 teaspoons of vanilla powder**
- **2 teaspoons of cinnamon**
- **4 cardamom capsules**
- **the juice and zest of 1 grated lemon**
- **2 teaspoons of agar-agar**

Clean the pumpkin, cut it into small pieces and make a puree that you will cook for 15 minutes with the juice and peel of the lemon and the cardamom seeds deprived of the shell. Continue cooking for another 20-30 minutes, mixing often and skimming if necessary. Add the chopped almonds, malt, cinnamon, and vanilla powder to the mixture. Mix well and add the agar-agar that you have previously dissolved in a little water and left to rest for at least 15 minutes. Continue to cook over high heat, stirring well for another 5 minutes, then put the jam in sterilized jars.

2) Lemon-scented apple jam

Ingredients:
- **1 kg of apples**
- **2 lemons**
- **2 tablespoons of 100% malt rice**
- **1 teaspoon of cinnamon**

Wash apples and lemons and dry them. Cut the apples into quarters without peeling them but removing only the core and seeds, then slice them very thinly. Cut the lemons with the peel into small pieces and remove all the seeds. Put the apples and lemons in a pot with the water and cook for 15 minutes over high heat. Lower the heat and continue cooking until the apple and lemons are crushed, forming a thick mixture. Use a puree or a mixer to blend the jam, then add the malt and cinnamon. Finally, raise the heat and finish cooking over high heat and stirring for a few minutes. Try the saucer test and keep. You can also decide to cook the lemons without the peel, adding the desired percentage of peel to the mixture just before potting.

3) Tofu sauce with pickles

Ingredients:
- **150 g of tofu**
- **200 g of mixed pickles**
- **the juice of ½ lemon**
- **water and salt to taste**

Blanch the pickles in boiling water to lose some of their vinegary flavors. Meanwhile, boil the tofu in a little salted water. Drain the pickles and make a fine beaten. Then blend the tofu with a bit of its cooking water. Add the chopped pickles to the tofu cream; season with lemon juice and salt. Mix evenly and serve.

4) Spicy pear jam

Ingredients:
- **1 kg of very sweet and ripe pears**
- **1 fresh hot pepper or 3 teaspoons of chili powder**
- **200 g of cane sugar**

Wash the pears, peel them, cut them into small pieces, and put them to cook in a pot with the freshly chopped chili or powder, adding a little water. Cook over medium heat, stirring more frequently when it reaches a boil. After about 30-40 minutes on the fire, the pears are almost entirely undone, and the mixture begins to thicken, losing all the remaining water. Then add the sugar, taking care to mix well so that the ingredients blend perfectly. Reached the right density, put the hot jam in hermetically sealed sterilized jars, turn them upside down on a wooden surface, cover them with a cloth and let them cool upside down until the vacuum is formed. Once opened, keep them in the refrigerator.

5) Autumn jam

Ingredients:
- **2 kg of peeled and boiled chestnuts**
- **5 large ripe apples**
- **100 g of raisins**
- **orange zest**
- **a few bay leaves and wild fennel**

Cook the chestnuts in plenty of lightly salted water, flavored with bay leaf and wild fennel. When they are well cooked, peel them, free them from the skin, and slice them. At the same time, wash and core and seed the apples, cut into small pieces. Also, prepare the orange peel cut finely and deprived of the white part. Mash the chestnuts well, put them in a pot with the apples, 1 cup of water, and part of the orange zest. Cook over high heat, using a flame-spreader net for an even distribution of heat until the apples are completely crushed. With the help of an immersion mixer, make a soft and not too dense compote; you can help yourself by adding more water or apple juice. Add the previously soaked raisins and the orange peel. Cook the jam for a few more minutes until it reaches the right density, and put it still hot. Sterilize the jars for extended storage.

6)   Grilled cherry tomato pesto, garlic, mint and hazelnuts

Ingredients:
- about 15 cherry tomatoes
- 1 handful of shelled hazelnuts
- 1 clove of garlic
- 1 teaspoon of dried mint
- extra virgin olive oil
- sea salt
- ½ teaspoon of turmeric powder

Wash the tomatoes, dry them and grill them whole on a plate or in the oven. As soon as the peel begins to color and break, mash them lightly with a spoon or fork. Continue cooking to brown them slightly. Finally, transfer them to a large bowl and let them cool slightly. Add the chopped hazelnuts more or less finely and the peeled and chopped garlic. Season with oil, salt, mint, and turmeric; finally, mash the mixture with a fork, mixing the ingredients well. If you don't eat it immediately, the pesto can be stored in the refrigerator, covered, for up to 2 days.

7)   Lentil ragout

Ingredients:
- 250 g of lentils
- 25 g of dried porcini mushrooms
- 1 stick of celery
- 1 carrot
- 1 small golden onion
- 1 bay leaf
- 1 tablespoon of tomato paste
- 500 g of tomato puree
- 1/2 glass of dry white wine
- 3 tablespoons of extra virgin olive oil
- 500 ml of hot water or vegetable broth
- salt
- pepper

To prepare the lentil ragout, first place the dried mushrooms in a bowl with warm water and leave them to soak for at least 30 minutes. In the meantime, clean the vegetables and chop them finely with a knife. Sauté them over low heat in a saucepan with a couple of tablespoons of oil. When they become translucent, add the drained, squeezed and finely chopped dried mushrooms and the bay leaf. Let it cook for 2 minutes, then add the rinsed lentils and sauté for a few minutes over medium heat. Add the white wine and let it evaporate. Add the tomato paste, puree, and hot water. Bring to a boil, add salt, pepper, cover and cook over low heat, as you would for the classic sauce for at least 1 hour and a half or 2, adding more hot water if necessary. At the end of cooking, the lentil sauce should be creamy and dense.

8) Eggplant pesto

Ingredients:
- 1 eggplant (about 350-400 g)
- 40 g of grated Parmesan
- 40 g of peeled and toasted almonds
- 1/2 clove of garlic (optional)
- 1 bunch of fresh basil
- extra virgin olive oil
- salt
- pepper

Wash the eggplant, dry it and pierce it with the tines of a fork. Place it on a baking sheet lined with parchment paper and cook it in a preheated oven at 200 ° for about 40-45 minutes or in any case until its pulp is soft. Remove from the oven and leave to cool. Remove the stalk, seeds, and skin and squeeze the remaining pulp. Transfer it to a bowl with the grated parmesan, basil, garlic, salt, pepper, toasted almonds. Blend everything with an immersion blender, adding the oil slowly until you get a cream of the desired consistency. Serve the eggplant pesto use it to season pasta.

9)   Guacamole

Ingredients:
- **Ripe avocado 1**
- **Green chilli 1**
- **Copper tomatoes 1**
- **Extra virgin olive oil 20 g**
- **Lime juice 10 g**
- **Shallot 10 g**
- **Black pepper 1 pinch**
- **Salt up to 1 pinch**

Start by looking after the avocado. Cut it in half lengthwise, then sink the knife's blade into the core and pull to extract it easily. Cut the pulp with a small knife to remove it more easily with a spoon; collect it in a small bowl. Then cut the lime in half and squeeze it to obtain the juice, be poured on the avocado pulp; Then, season with salt and pepper, and mash the pulp with a fork. Set aside, then peel and finely chop the shallot, then wash, dry, and slice the tomato: obtained from the cubes' slices. Then tick the green (or red) chili pepper, empty it of its seeds, cut it into strips, and then into cubes. Then in the bowl with the crushed avocado pulp, pour the chopped shallot and the diced tomatoes. Also, add the chili and oil, stir and add more salt and pepper if necessary. Your guacamole sauce is ready to be enjoyed!

10) Fresh tomato sauce with basil

Ingredients:
- **Copper tomatoes 1.2 kg**
- **Extra virgin olive oil 3 tbsp**
- **Salt up to taste**
- **Basil 8 leaves**

Remove the stalks and wash them very well, then dry them. Cut each tomato into two halves and remove the green part of each of them' stem. Squeeze the two halves of the tomato into a bowl or sink so that all the seeds come out. Put the tomatoes in a steel pot, which you will arrange on low heat covered by the lid; let the tomatoes cook, turning them from time to time until they are wilted and come apart. Pass the tomatoes with a vegetable mill making the sauce converge in a bowl; once all the tomatoes have been passed, pour the sauce into a smaller steel pot that you will put on the stove. Add the salt and oil to the sauce, consume it over high heat to the desired density, turn off the heat, and add the whole basil or coarsely chopped by hand. Perfect with spaghetti!

11) Tuna sauce

Ingredients:

- **100 g of tuna in oil**
- **50 g of pickled capers**
- **2 anchovies**
- **1 firm yolk**
- **the juice of 1/2 lemon**
- **1 glass of extra virgin olive oil**
- **salt**
- **pepper**

To make the tuna sauce, start chopping the tuna well drained from the oil and collect it in the mixing bowl together with the rinsed and squeezed capers, the boned anchovies, and the crumbled hard-boiled egg yolk. Soften the dough with a few tablespoons of oil and operate the appliance with short interrupted clicks. Gradually add the rest of the oil and blend for a few seconds until the desired density is obtained. Add the lemon juice filtered through a colander and mix very well. Taste and, if necessary, season with salt and pepper. Let it sit for 10 minutes. If the sauce is too thick, dilute it with a little oil. Then pour the tuna sauce in a gravy boat or a serving bowl and serve.

12) Pear and cinnamon sauce

Ingredients:
- **Pears (pulp) 500 g**
- **Ground cinnamon ½ tsp**
- **Sugar 100 g**
- **½ glass white wine**
- **Lemon juice 1 tbsp**

Wash, peel, cut into quarters, and core the pears. Cut the pulp into small pieces and place it in a saucepan in which you will add the wine, sugar, cinnamon, and lemon juice. Bring everything slowly to a boil, and, keeping the heat low, cook and thicken the mixture (about 20-25 minutes). Turn off the heat and let it cool, then pass the mixture to the mixer before using.

13) Milk cream

Ingredients:
- **Whole milk 400 g**
- **Honey 1 tsp**
- **Sugar 80 g**
- **Vanilla bean 1**
- **Corn starch 40 g**
- **Fresh liquid cream 150 g**

Heat 300 g of milk with the sugar in a saucepan. Cut the vanilla bean lengthwise, extract the seeds, scrap it with a small knife; add the seeds of the vanilla bean in the milk and heat over very low heat, and mix well with the whisk to dissolve the sugar. In a separate bowl, sift the corn starch, then pour the remaining milk, mixing with a hand whisk: by doing so, you will avoid the formation of lumps in the cream. Add the cold milk in which the corn starch has dissolved into the saucepan with the milk and sugar. Also, add the honey, continuing with the whisk always on very low heat until the cream has thickened. Once it is thick and homogeneous, turn off and pour the cream you have obtained into a bowl. Cover with the transparent film in contact, making it adhere well to the surface so that the annoying crust does not form; let it cool to room temperature and then refrigerate. After the necessary time has elapsed, remove the cream from the refrigerator: if you find any lumps, sift it with a fine mesh strainer to eliminate them. Heat the cream with an electric mixer, then whip the cold cream from the refrigerator in a separate bowl. Add the whipped cream to the now cold milk cream, mixing the two compounds very gently from bottom to top until a smooth and homogeneous cream is obtained. Your milk cream is ready: you can use it to fill cream puffs, biscuit dough rolls, cakes, and other desserts!

<h1 align="center">14) Lemon cream</h1>

Ingredients:

- **Whole milk 500 ml**
- **Sugar 150 g**
- **Potato starch 35 g**
- **00 flour 35 g**
- **Yolks 6**
- **Lemon zest 3**

Take the zest of the lemons taking care not to get the white part, and pour the zest into a pan where you have added the milk. Turn on the low heat and let the milk cool. Meanwhile, in a bowl, place the egg yolks, sugar and work the mixture with a whisk. You will need to obtain a homogeneous cream before adding the sifted flour and starch; mix with a whisk to mix the powders, then add the warmed milk. Stir vigorously to obtain a homogeneous and fluid mixture, then pour it back into the pan, filtering it with a fine mesh strainer to prevent lumps from forming. Turn on the low heat and cook the cream, continually stirring with the whisk, until it has thickened (it will take about 15 minutes). When it has reduced, before turning off the heat, you can grate the zest of lemon if you prefer to flavor it more; then turn off the heat and transfer the cream into a bowl, then cover it with the cling film and let it cool before putting it back in the fridge and being able to use it!

15) Black olives patè

Ingredients:
- **Black olives 200 g**
- **Extra virgin olive oil 45 g**

To prepare the olive pate, start by pitting the olives one by one, put them in the blender, and blend them until you get a homogeneous mixture. Add the oil dropwise to the extra virgin olive oil until you get a soft and sufficiently compact cream. Your pate is ready to be served. You can enjoy it on crunchy croutons: to prepare them, slice the bread, place it on a dripping pan lined with baking paper, sprinkle it with a drizzle of oil, and toast it on the oven in grill mode for 2 minutes, turning it halfway through cooking to toast it. Evenly. You can spread the black olive pate on warm bread with a drizzle of oil cooked in the oven until it takes on a golden color.

Conclusion

20% of people in the developed world suffer from eczema: the rate of accidents between infants and children increases. Research shows eczema sufferers spend up to $ 1,000 on eczema treatments each year, and nearly 40% spend more than 10 minutes each day applying topical treatments. Yet, the number of people with eczema is on the rise and has tripled in recent years. While it is perfectly okay to use modern medications to help you or your child get temporary relief, a long-term solution should be explored and ultimately followed. This solution involves making environmental and dietary changes. This exceptional program offers solutions and advice that can be tailored to your own needs; eventually, you will manage eczema.